C000016037

Tess Connors

PALEO DIET

FOR FAMILY

3 BOOKS IN 1

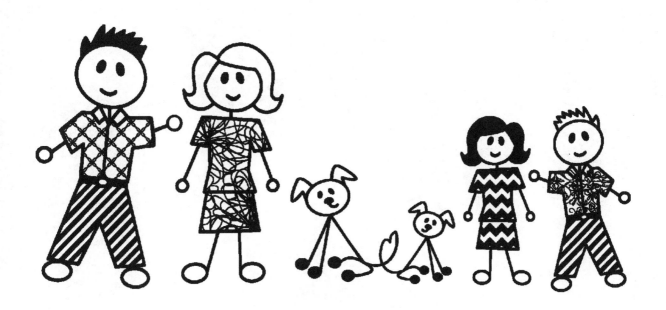

Copyright 2021 – All rights reserved.

The content contained within this book may not be reproduced, duplicated or transmitted without direct written permission from the author or the publisher.

Under no circumstances will any blame or legal responsibility be held against the publisher, or author, for any damages, reparation, or monetary loss due to the information contained within this book. Either directly or indirectly.

Legal Notice:

This book is copyright protected. This book is only for personal use. You cannot amend, distribute, sell, use, quote or paraphrase any part, or the content within this book, without the consent of the author or publisher.

Disclaimer Notice:

Please note the information contained within this document is for educational and entertainment purposes only. All effort has been executed to present accurate, up to date, and reliable, complete information. No warranties of any kind are declared or implied. Readers acknowledge that the author is not engaging in the rendering of legal, financial, medical or professional advice. The content within this book has been derived from various sources. Please consult a licensed professional before attempting any techniques outlined in this book.

By reading this document, the reader agrees that under no circumstances is the author responsible for any losses, direct or indirect, which are incurred as a result of the use of information contained within this document, including, but not limited to, — errors, omissions, or inaccuracies.

Table of Contents:

INTRODUCTION

Paleo-diet, also known as paleolithic diet or cave diet, **is a contemporary diet which would like to propose a hypothetical type of nutrition which would have characterized human populations lived in the period preceding the introduction of agriculture, about 10,000 years ago**.

The diet was developed for the first time in the '30s by dentist Weston A. Price who, after his travels around the world, became convinced that in some primitive populations the absence of some diseases, such as caries and tuberculosis, was attributable to the diet they followed.

What are the benefits of paleodiet for your family?

✓ More health,
✓ Less fat,
✓ Less cellulite;

Mass overweight is a modern problem, unknown in the paleolithic era. The watchword of the paleo diet: "natural."

Our ancestors ate what they found available to them: berries and fruits, vegetables, hunted meat, caught fish and no refined flours and no sweets. Junk foods and industrial products were not a threat, they simply didn't exist.

This style of eating is not so much about counting calories, nor does it prescribe specific amounts of food, but it still helps you lose weight. The secret is soon told: it is a real lifestyle that aims to get closer to the true nature of man, for whom physical exercise is essential, to build lean mass with constant walks in the open air during daylight hours, because the current life leads to a desynchronization of our biological clock compared to the rhythms of nature. Eating like the primitives means understanding what are the balances that have kept our species alive for millions of years without drugs, and try to bring us back, as far as possible, to that style.

Reactivates the metabolism and satiates you faster!

The paleo diet makes you slim because it causes a reduction in the body's inflammatory state, which brings with it a reactivation of the metabolism. Natural foods nourish with fewer calories and have greater cleansing power. According to the paleo diet, our body is made to use as energy sources also fats and proteins, foods that quickly trigger the stop of hunger. The modern diet, instead, rich in carbohydrates, bypasses these mechanisms. That's why it's easy to overdo eating bread and pasta: our body is not predisposed to say "stop" to these foods.

But how did the paleolithic people eat? Meat, fish and eggs are allowed, while cereals, milk and derivatives, legumes and industrial sugars are to be avoided. If meat must be, it must come from animals fed in a natural way, such as cattle with grass, fish must not be farmed, eggs from chickens and seasonal vegetables, zero kilometer, grown without pesticides. The benefits? Greater presence of slimming nutrients in what we eat: more vitamins, more antioxidants, more good fats, all valuable metabolic activators.

Important:
To lose weight, however, you need to combine your diet with exercise, such as walking, going to the gym, biking and more. This cookbook lists a number of Paleo recipes that are not intended to replace the advice of a nutritionist.

MEASUREMENT CONVERSION

Volume Equivalents (Liquid)

Type	US Standard (ounces)	Metric
2 tablespoons	1 fl. oz.	30 mL
¼ cup	2 fl. oz.	60 mL
½ cup	4 fl. oz.	120 mL
1 cup	8 fl. oz.	240mL

Volume Equivalents (Dry)

Type	Metric
¼ teaspoon	1 mL
½ teaspoon	2 mL
1 teaspoon	5 mL
1 tablespoon	15 mL
¼ cup	59 mL
½ cup	118 mL
1 cup	235 mL

Oven Temperatures

Fahrenheit (°F)	Celsius (°C)
250	120
300	150
325	165
350	180
375	190
400	200
425	220
450	230

THE 10 GOLDEN RULES

1. Keep 10 Paleo foods on hand at all times, in your office, in your home, in your car, in your wallet. Nuts and pumpkin seeds are great options.
2. Plan a menu of meals for the week. This will help you know what to buy at the grocery store and ensure you have a delicious, healthy meal every day.
3. Cook large portions. This will help you have ready, healthy food on hand for a couple of days.
4. Don't keep foods in the house that are not paleo friendly. If this will be on hand, it will be a great temptation.
5. If you find it hard to eliminate some foods that you have a sweet tooth for that aren't 100% paleo, start decreasing the portions.
6. Don't run out of food. Can't cook anything? Don't have anything paleo at home to eat that's healthy? Are you hungry? Don't let this happen to you, it's very easy in these cases to give in to temptation.
7. Try new ingredients and seasonings. Seasonings are great for improving the taste of a dish and trying new innovative dishes.
8. If possible, freeze some of the foods you've cooked. This way, you have something on hand in the freezer, so if you don't have time to go grocery shopping, you won't starve.
9. Fall in love with plants, which are essential to your health and fitness. Don't be afraid to try new vegetables in different colors.
10. Avoid cooking the same things over and over again, you'll end up bored with your diet.

<u>Enjoy the paleo diet and all your meals!</u>

BOOK 1

PALEO DIET FOR MEN

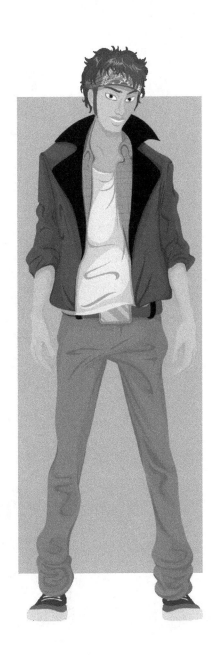

BLACK ONION RELISH

Serv.: 4 | **Prep.:** 10m | **Cook:** 35m

Ingredients:
- ✓ 2 yellow onions
- ✓ 1 red bell pepper, chopped
- ✓ 2 tablespoons chopped fresh flat-leaf parsley
- ✓ Salt and freshly ground black pepper to taste
- ✓ 1 pinch cayenne pepper, or more to taste
- ✓ 3 tablespoons sherry vinegar
- ✓ 3 tablespoons olive oil

Directions: Prepare a charcoal grill or make a campfire and let the fire burn until it has accumulated a bed of coals.
Nestle the onions into the hot area. Pile up the coals on the sides and top. Roast the onions for 15 minutes until tender and blackened. Flip the onions and rebury them. Cook for 10-15 more minutes until the onions start to leak juice. To check, insert a bamboo skewer into the center and see if it slides in so easily. Transfer the onions into the bowl. Cover the bowl and let them cool.
Arrange the red pepper into the coals and cook for 10 minutes, flipping frequently until charred.
Peel and remove the blackened skin of the onions. Scrape off the charred black portions of the red pepper. Chop both red pepper and onions finely. Mix them in a bowl together with the parsley. Season the mixture with black pepper, cayenne pepper, and salt according to your taste.
Toss in olive oil and sherry vinegar with the relish. Cover, refrigerate it for 1 hour.

BLACK SESAME SEED AND WALNUT MIX

Serv.: 24 | **Prep.:** 5m | **Cook:** 10m

Ingredients:
- ✓ 2 cups black sesame seeds
- ✓ 2 cups walnut pieces

Directions: In a big skillet, cook and stir the sesame seeds on medium heat until seeds begin to pop and smell toasted, for about 7 minutes. While toasting sesame seeds, microwave the walnuts for about 2 minutes, until tangy. Let walnuts and sesame seeds cool to room temperature. When cooled, put walnuts and sesame seeds in a blender. Blend until finely ground. Keep in an airtight container, put in fridge for storage.

BLACKENED CHICKEN

Serv.: 2 | **Prep.:** 10m | **Cook:** 10m

Ingredients:
- ✓ 1/2 teaspoon paprika
- ✓ 1/8 teaspoon salt
- ✓ 1/4 teaspoon cayenne pepper
- ✓ 1/4 teaspoon ground cumin
- ✓ 1/4 teaspoon dried thyme
- ✓ 1/8 teaspoon ground white pepper
- ✓ 1/8 teaspoon onion powder
- ✓ 2 skinless, boneless chicken breast halves

Directions: Prepare the oven by heating to 350°F or 175°C. Apply a bit of grease to a baking sheet. Heat a cast-iron skillet until piping hot on high heat. Combine onion powder, white pepper, paprika, cayenne, salt, cumin and thyme. Apply cooking spray on the chicken breasts on both sides then coat with spice mixture.
Put the chicken breasts in a hot pan and cook for about a minute on each side. Then, transfer the chicken to the baking sheet.
Let it bake in the oven and cook the chicken for five minutes or until it is not pink.

BLUEBERRY SALSA

Serv.: 24 | **Prep.:** 15m | **Cook:** 0

Ingredients:
- ✓ 2 cups chopped fresh blueberries
- ✓ 1 cup whole fresh blueberries
- ✓ 1 tablespoon finely chopped jalapeno pepper
- ✓ 1/3 cup chopped red onion
- ✓ 1/4 cup chopped red bell pepper
- ✓ 1 fresh lime, juiced
- ✓ Salt to taste

Directions: Mix together salt, lime juice, red pepper, onion, jalapeno pepper, chopped and whole blueberries in a bowl.

BOILED LOBSTER

Serv.: 2| **Prep.:** 30m | **Cook:** 15m

Ingredients:
- ✓ 3 gallons water
- ✓ 2 large onions, quartered
- ✓ 10 cloves garlic, peeled and cut in half
- ✓ 2 lemons, quartered
- ✓ 2 oranges, quartered
- ✓ 5 stalks celery, quartered
- ✓ 4 tablespoons black pepper
- ✓ 4 tablespoons seasoned salt
- ✓ 6 fresh jalapeno peppers (optional)
- ✓ 2 fresh live lobsters

Directions: Into a large pot, add water and then add jalapeno peppers, onions, seasoned salt, garlic, black pepper, lemons, celery and oranges. Heat to a full rolling boil and let it boil for about 20 minutes.
Place in lobsters and cover the pot with a lid. Let it boil for about 15 minutes (depends on the size of lobsters). Take the lobsters out of the pot and put in a colander under cool running water to finish cooking and then serve.

BOSS PIZZA SAUCE

Serv.: 12| **Prep.:** 10m | **Cook:** 0

Ingredients:
- ✓ 1 (15 ounce) can low-sodium tomato sauce
- ✓ 1 (6 ounce) can low-sodium tomato paste
- ✓ 2 teaspoons ground black pepper
- ✓ 1 1/2 teaspoons dried oregano
- ✓ 1/2 teaspoon dried basil leaves
- ✓ 1/2 teaspoon garlic powder
- ✓ 1 1/2 teaspoons salt
- ✓ 1/4 teaspoon dried thyme leaves
- ✓ 1/4 teaspoon dried cilantro
- ✓ 1/4 teaspoon dried parsley
- ✓ 1/4 teaspoon onion salt

Directions: In a bowl, combine together onion salt, parsley, cilantro, thyme, salt, garlic powder, basil, oregano, ground black pepper, tomato paste and tomato sauce until well blended.

BRAISED BALSAMIC CHICKEN

Serv.: 6| **Prep.:** 10m | **Cook:** 25m

Ingredients:
- ✓ 6 skinless, boneless chicken breast halves
- ✓ 1 teaspoon garlic salt
- ✓ Ground black pepper to taste
- ✓ 2 tablespoons olive oil
- ✓ 1 onion, thinly sliced
- ✓ 1 (14.5 ounce) can diced tomatoes
- ✓ 1/2 cup balsamic vinegar
- ✓ 1 teaspoon dried basil
- ✓ 1 teaspoon dried oregano
- ✓ 1 teaspoon dried rosemary
- ✓ 1/2 teaspoon dried thyme

Directions: Use pepper and garlic salt to season both sides of chicken breasts.
In a skillet over medium heat, put in oil then heat it; add seasoned chicken breasts and cook for 3-4 minutes per side until chicken turns brown. Put in onion; stir and cook for 3-4 minutes until onion turns brown.
Pour balsamic vinegar and diced tomatoes over chicken; use thyme, rosemary, oregano, and basil for seasoning. Simmer for about 15 minutes until the juices run clear and chicken is not pink anymore. An instant-read thermometer inserted into the center should register at least 165 degrees F (74 degrees C).

BRAZILIAN CHICKEN WITH COCONUT MILK

Serv.: 4 | **Prep.:** 15m | **Cook:** 15m

Ingredients:
- ✓ 1 teaspoon ground cumin
- ✓ 1 teaspoon ground cayenne pepper

- ✓ 1 teaspoon ground turmeric
- ✓ 1 teaspoon ground coriander
- ✓ 4 skinless, boneless chicken breast halves
- ✓ Salt and pepper to taste
- ✓ 2 tablespoons olive oil
- ✓ 1 onion, chopped
- ✓ 1 tablespoon minced fresh ginger
- ✓ 2 jalapeno peppers, seeded and chopped
- ✓ 2 cloves garlic, minced
- ✓ 3 tomatoes, seeded and chopped
- ✓ 1 (14 ounce) can light coconut milk
- ✓ 1 bunch chopped fresh parsley

Directions: Mix together coriander, turmeric, cayenne pepper, and cumin in a medium bowl. Add in the chicken and season with salt and pepper. Rub spice mixture thoroughly on all sides.
In a skillet, heat 1 tablespoon of olive oil over medium heat. Transfer chicken to the skillet. Cook until juices are clear and chicken is no longer pink, for 10 to 15 minutes per side. Transfer chicken off heat and set aside.
In the skillet, heat remaining olive oil. Stir in garlic, jalapeno peppers, ginger, and onions and cook until tender for 5 minutes. Mix tomatoes in and cook for 5 to 8 minutes. Stir coconut milk in. Pour over chicken and serve with garnished parsley.

BRAZILIAN CHURRASCO

Serv.: 2 | **Prep.:** 5m | **Cook:** 10m

Ingredients:
- ✓ 1 (12 ounce) 1/2-inch thick top sirloin steak
- ✓ Sea salt (such as Morton's®) to taste

Directions: Rub the sirloin steak using sea salt while pressing until the steak is evenly coated and the salt sticks on each side.
Preheat the grill over medium heat and coat the grate lightly with oil.
Cook the steak on the grill for about 5 minutes until browned. Turn the steak and then scrape off as much salt as you can at the top. Continue to cook for 5 to 10 minutes until second side turns brown and the center reaches the doneness desired.
Scrape off salt on the second side and then serve.

BREAKFAST ZINGER JUICE

Serv.: 2 | **Prep.:** 5m | **Cook:** 0

Ingredients:
- ✓ 2 lemons - peeled, seeded, and quartered
- ✓ 2 carrots, chopped
- ✓ 2 apples, quartered
- ✓ 2 beets, trimmed and chopped

Directions: Press beets, apples, carrots and lemons through a juicer and into a big glass.

EGGPLANT IN COCONUT MILK

Serv.: 6 | **Prep.:** 15m | **Cook:** 17m

Ingredients:
- ✓ 2 large brinjal (eggplant), sliced
- ✓ 1/4 teaspoon chile powder, or more to taste
- ✓ 1/8 teaspoon turmeric powder, or more to taste
- ✓ 1 tablespoon vegetable oil, or more as needed
- ✓ Salt to taste
- ✓ 1 cup coconut milk, or more to taste
- ✓ 2 tablespoons tamarind pulp, juice squeezed
- ✓ 1 1/2 tablespoons chile powder
- ✓ 1 tablespoon coriander powder
- ✓ 1/2 teaspoon turmeric powder
- ✓ For Tempering:
- ✓ 2 tablespoons vegetable oil
- ✓ 1 teaspoon mustard seed
- ✓ 1 sprig fresh curry leaves
- ✓ 2 dried red chile peppers

Directions: Season brinjal with salt, 1/8 tsp. turmeric powder, and 1/4 tsp. chile powder. Put aside for 3-4 minutes to set flavors.
In a big skillet, heat 1 tbsp. oil on medium heat. Stir and cook brinjal for 10 minutes until tender and lightly browned. Take off heat.
In a saucepan mix 1/2 tsp. turmeric powder, coriander powder, 1 1/2 tbsp. chile powder, reserved tamarind juice, and coconut milk. Heat on medium heat for 5-10 minutes to merge flavors. Mix in cooked brinjal and stir well.
In another skillet, heat 2 tbsp. vegetable oil on medium heat. Stir and cook dried chile peppers,

curry leaves, and mustard seed for 2-3 minutes until toasted and fragrant. Put oil mixture on brinjal.

BROCCOLI IN ROAST CHICKEN DRIPPINGS

Serv.: 4 | **Prep.:** 5m | **Cook:** 10m

Ingredients:
- ✓ 1/4 cup roast chicken drippings
- ✓ 1 head broccoli, cut into florets
- ✓ 2 cloves garlic, chopped

Directions: Take the roasted chicken out of the roasting pan and put in on a serving tray to rest after having roasted. Leave the oven on. Pour off the excess drippings from the roasting pan and save enough just to coat the broccoli. Toss together garlic and broccoli in the drippings until coated well and put in the still hot oven. Roast until tender, for 5-8 minutes.

MACKEREL FILLET WITH PAPRIKA

Serv.: 6 | **Prep.:** 10m | **Cook:** 5m

Ingredients:
- ✓ 6 (3 ounce) fillets Spanish mackerel fillets
- ✓ 1/4 cup olive oil
- ✓ 1/2 teaspoon paprika
- ✓ Salt and ground black pepper to taste
- ✓ 12 slices lemon

Directions: Preheat oven broiler. Put oven rack about 6-in. away from heat source. Grease a baking dish lightly. Rub each side of every mackerel fillet using olive oil. Put on prepped baking dish, skin side down. Season with pepper, salt and paprika. Put 2 lemon slices on every fillet.
Bake fillets for 5-7 minutes under the broiler until fish just starts to flake. Immediately serve.

BROILED SUMMER SQUASH WITH RADISH

Serv.: 4 | **Prep.:** 20m | **Cook:** 20m

Ingredients:
- ✓ 1/4 cup extra virgin olive oil
- ✓ 1/4 cup balsamic vinegar
- ✓ 1 teaspoon chopped fresh dill
- ✓ 1/4 teaspoon salt
- ✓ 1/2 teaspoon freshly cracked black pepper
- ✓ 1/2 cup chopped red onion
- ✓ 1 large zucchini, cut in half lengthwise then into 1/4-inch slices
- ✓ 1 large yellow squash, cut into 1/2-inch cubes
- ✓ 4 radishes, cut into 1/4-inch-thick slices

Directions: Start preheating the oven's broiler and place oven rack in a 6"-distance away from the heat.
In a mixing bowl, combine pepper, salt, dill, vinegar and olive oil until incorporated. Put in radishes, yellow squash, zucchini and onion; toss to coat evenly. Transfer to an 8x8" baking dish, wrap aluminum foil over the top.
Broil in prepared oven for 10 minutes, removing foil, and keep broiling for another 10 minutes until vegetables are softened and browned evenly on top.

SALAD DRESSING

Serv.: 16 | **Prep.:** 10m | **Cook:** 0

Ingredients:
- ✓ 1/2 cup rice vinegar
- ✓ 2 tablespoons red wine vinegar
- ✓ 2 tablespoons honey
- ✓ 1 tablespoon sesame oil
- ✓ 1 teaspoon dried rosemary
- ✓ 1 teaspoon dried basil
- ✓ 1 teaspoon dried marjoram
- ✓ 1 teaspoon dry mustard powder
- ✓ 3 cloves garlic, pressed
- ✓ Salt and pepper to taste
- ✓ 1 cup vegetable oil

Directions: In a bowl, combine pepper, salt, garlic, mustard, marjoram, basil, rosemary, sesame oil, honey, red wine vinegar, and rice vinegar until blended. Mix in vegetable oil, and then add to a vinaigrette shaker. Before serving, chill overnight for the flavors to combine. Shake to blend before pouring.

CABBAGE WITH LIME

Serv.: 20| **Prep.:** 20m | **Cook:** 0

Ingredients:
- ✓ 1 medium head cabbage, chopped
- ✓ 6 Roma (plum) tomatoes, diced
- ✓ 1 red onion, diced
- ✓ 1 yellow onion, diced
- ✓ 4 jalapeno peppers, diced
- ✓ 2 bunches cilantro, chopped
- ✓ 3 limes, juiced
- ✓ 2 teaspoons chopped garlic
- ✓ 2 teaspoons salt

Directions: In a big bowl, combine together salt, garlic, lime juice, cilantro, jalapeno pepper, yellow onion, red onion, tomatoes and cabbage.
Use plastic wrap to cover bowl and chill for a minimum of 2 hours.

CABBAGE STEAKS

Serv.: 6| **Prep.:** 15m | **Cook:** 45m

Ingredients:
- ✓ 1 head cabbage
- ✓ 2 tablespoons light olive oil
- ✓ 2 tablespoons minced garlic
- ✓ 1/2 teaspoon salt, or to taste
- ✓ 1/2 teaspoon ground black pepper, or to taste

Directions: Set the oven to 175°C or 350°F to preheat.
Cut off the bottom of the cabbage and set it to let the flat end lay on the cutting board, then slice into pieces with the thickness of 1 inch. Spread the slices in a big casserole dish in a single layer.
Pour over the cabbage slices with olive oil and put garlic on top. Season with pepper and salt, then use aluminum foil to cover the dish.
In the preheated oven, bake for 45 minutes, until you can pierce the cabbage core easily with a fork.

CAJUN PRIME RIB

Serv.: 6| **Prep.:** 15m | **Cook:** 45m

Ingredients:
- ✓ 1 (7 pound) 3 rib prime rib beef roast
- ✓ 1/4 cup black pepper
- ✓ 1/4 cup garlic powder
- ✓ 1/4 cup salt
- ✓ 1 large onion, sliced
- ✓ 1 pound sliced bacon
- ✓ 1 tablespoon Cajun seasoning, or to taste

Directions: Gently cut the fat cap on top of the prime rib roast, being cautious not to slice into the meat. Reserve the fat. Cover the roast completely with black pepper, then garlic powder, then with. Arrange sliced onion on top of salt to cover. Secure some onion with toothpicks. Place the fat cap over the onions, securing into the roast with toothpicks. Add bacon on top of the onions, securing with toothpicks as well. Wrap tightly in aluminum foil and store in the refrigerator overnight.
Preheat the oven to 285°C (550°F) the next morning. Remove the foil from the roast and prick with a knife a few times. Cover with foil again and put in a shallow baking dish.
Roast in the heated oven for 35 minutes. Take out from the oven and let it cool slightly, not longer than half an hour. Store in the refrigerator for a minimum of 3 hours.
Preheat a grill over high heat. Take out the fat cap and bacon and take off the seasoning and onions. Slice the roast using a sharp knife into steaks. Every rib will yield 2 steaks, one with bone and one without. Sprinkle steaks with Cajun seasoning with your desired amount. You may grill bacon or reserve for other use.
Slightly oil the grill grate. Grill steaks to your desired doneness.

CAJUN SPICED PORK CHOPS

Serv.: 4| **Prep.:** 5m | **Cook:** 10m

Ingredients:
- ✓ 1 teaspoon paprika

- ✓ 1/2 teaspoon ground cumin
- ✓ 1/2 teaspoon ground black pepper
- ✓ 1/2 teaspoon cayenne pepper
- ✓ 1/2 teaspoon rubbed dried sage leaves
- ✓ 1/2 teaspoon garlic salt
- ✓ 1 1/2 teaspoons extra-virgin olive oil
- ✓ 4 center cut pork chops

Directions: On a plate, combine garlic salt, sage, cayenne pepper, black pepper, cumin and paprika. Use a generous amount of spice mixture to coat each pork chop.

In a large skillet over high heat, heat several pumps of butter-flavored, non-stick spray and olive oil. Put the pork chops into the skillet, lowering the heat to medium. Cook the pork for 8-10 minutes until the center is no longer pink. An instant-read thermometer should read 145°F (63°C) when inserted into the center.

CALAMARI SALAD

Serv.: 8| **Prep.:** 15m | **Cook:** 10m

Ingredients:
- ✓ 1/2 cup olive oil
- ✓ 1/4 cup red wine vinegar
- ✓ 2 cloves garlic, pressed
- ✓ 1 cup dry white wine
- ✓ 1 cup water
- ✓ 1 pound squid, cleaned and cut into rings and tentacles
- ✓ 1 cup chopped celery
- ✓ 1/2 bunch chopped fresh cilantro
- ✓ 1 green bell pepper, chopped
- ✓ 1 red bell pepper, chopped
- ✓ 1 yellow bell pepper, chopped
- ✓ 1 cup chopped cucumber
- ✓ 1 bunch fresh green onions, chopped
- ✓ 1 bunch chopped fresh parsley
- ✓ 1 cup jicama, peeled and shredded
- ✓ 1 jalapeno pepper, finely chopped

Directions: Mix garlic, red wine vinegar, and olive oil in a small bowl.

Put wine and water on a low boil in a medium saucepan. Mix in the squid and cook for about 2 minutes until opaque. Drain then cool.

In a big bowl. Stir jalapeno, jicama, parsley, green onions, cucumber, cilantro, celery, and yellow, red, and green bell pepper. Gently toss with squid and olive oil dressing mixture. Chill prior to serving.

CALVES LIVER WITH LEMON THYME

Serv.: 2| **Prep.:** 7m | **Cook:** 8m

Ingredients:
- ✓ 8 ounces calves liver, sliced
- ✓ 1 tablespoon olive oil
- ✓ 6 sprigs fresh lemon thyme, chopped
- ✓ Salt and pepper to taste

Directions: Rinse the liver under running water and pat dry. On medium heat, pour oil in a big non-stick pan and heat. Layer fresh thyme in the bottom of the pan and top with the liver. Cook for 4-5 minutes per side on medium heat. The calves' liver can be consumed even if a little pink, but make sure not to overcook it. Once done cooking, sprinkle pepper and salt to season.

CANDIED BACON AND CURRY CASHEW MIX

Serv.: 2| **Prep.:** 10m | **Cook:** 14m

Ingredients:
- ✓ 1/3 cup chopped bacon
- ✓ 1 tablespoon raw sugar
- ✓ 1 1/2 tablespoons olive oil
- ✓ 1/2 cup roasted and salted whole cashews
- ✓ 1 tablespoon yellow curry powder
- ✓ 1 teaspoon garlic powder

Directions: Heat a skillet on medium-high heat. Stir and cook the bacon and sugar. Cook for 10 minutes until the sugar starts caramelizing, and the bacon is crispy. Then remove from the heat.

In a separate pan, heat olive oil on medium-high. Add the cashews, garlic powder, and curry powder. Stir and cook for 4-5 minutes until heated and aromatic.

In a bowl, mix the seasoned cashews and bacon.

Chicken & Orange

Serv.: 4 | **Prep.:** 10m | **Cook:** 10m

Ingredients:
- ✓ 4 skinless, boneless chicken breast halves - pounded thin
- ✓ 6 oranges, juiced
- ✓ 3 tablespoons thinly sliced green onion
- ✓ Ground black pepper to taste

Directions: Using a tenderizing mallet, hit the chicken fillets until they are a bit thinned out. Put the black pepper, green onions and orange juice into a frying pan on medium heat. Don't cook on high heat because the juice might burn and get bitter.
Poach the chicken in the juice mixture until the juices run clear and becomes firm. This will take approximately 10 minutes; it depends on the thickness of the fillets. Put the chicken on a serving plate and pour some of the juice mixture on top, then serve.

Cashew Butter

Serv.: 34 | **Prep.:** 15m | **Cook:** 0

Ingredients:
- ✓ 3 cups unsalted cashews (such as Stock Barrel®), divided
- ✓ 1/3 cup vegetable oil, or more as needed
- ✓ 1 teaspoon sea salt

Directions: While drizzling vegetable oil in mixture to make it move, process 1 cup cashews in bowl of food processor. Alternating with oil, put cashews in food processor; process. Add sea salt when all cashews are added; process for 10-15 minutes till you get preferred texture.

Cassava Flour Shortbread Cookies

Serv.: 36 | **Prep.:** 15m | **Cook:** 12m

Ingredients:
- ✓ 1/2 cup grass-fed butter, softened
- ✓ 1/3 cup maple syrup
- ✓ 1 teaspoon vanilla extract
- ✓ 1 1/2 cups cassava flour (such as Otto's®)
- ✓ 1/4 teaspoon salt

Directions: Mix vanilla, maple syrup and butter together in a bowl of stand mixer with paddle attached; beat until a creamy and smooth mixture is formed. Put in salt and flour; keep mixing until it forms into a tough dough. Press dough down into a disc to flatten, cover with plastic wrap, then chill for half an hour.
Set oven to 175°C (or 350°F) and begin preheating. Prepare two parchment-lined baking sheets.
Place dough between 2 parchment paper sheets and roll into 1/4" pieces. Use cookie cutters to cut out shape; arrange the cut-out dough in a 2"-distance away from each other on lined baking sheets.
Bake for 12-14 minutes in the prepared oven until edges are golden. Allow to chill on the sheet for 60 seconds, then move to a wire rack to cool thoroughly.

Cassava Flour Pita Chips

Serv.: 4 | **Prep.:** 20m | **Cook:** 15m

Ingredients:
- ✓ 3/4 cup warm water (100 to 105 degrees F/38 to 41 degrees C)
- ✓ 3/4 teaspoon coconut sugar
- ✓ 3/4 teaspoon active dry yeast
- ✓ 1 1/2 teaspoons olive oil (such as Kasandrino's®)
- ✓ 1/2 teaspoon sea salt (such as Redmond® Real Salt)
- ✓ 1/4 teaspoon Italian seasoning (optional)
- ✓ 2/3 cup cassava flour (such as Otto's®), or more as needed
- ✓ 1/4 cup arrowroot starch
- ✓ 3/4 teaspoon unflavored gelatin
- ✓ 1 tablespoon arrowroot starch, or as needed

Directions: Start preheating oven to 230 degrees C

(450 degrees F). Prepare a parchment paper-lined baking sheet.

In a large glass measuring cup, mix warm water, yeast and coconut sugar; allow to stand for 4 to 6 minutes until yeast softens and a creamy foam starts to form. Stir in olive oil, Italian seasoning and sea salt.

In a bowl, beat together cassava flour, gelatin and 1/4 cup arrowroot starch; add into the yeast mixture and stir using a wooden spoon. If dough is too sticky, add a few tablespoons of cassava flour several at a time. Separate into 4 parts and form into balls then gently knead each one.

Dust 1/4 tablespoon arrowroot starch onto a piece of parchment paper and put 1 dough ball on it. Sprinkle with more arrowroot and place on top a second piece of parchment. Shape dough into a 4-inch circle. For crisper pita chips, roll it to a 5-inch circle. Place the dough on the prepared baking sheet. Do the same with remaining dough and arrowroot starch.

In preheated oven, bake for 5 minutes. Take out of oven and carefully slice each circle into 8 wedges. Place in the oven and bake for 5 minutes longer. Turnover each wedge and bake for 5 to 8 minutes, until chips are crisp and edges are golden.

CAULIFLOWER EGGPLANT CURRY CUMIN ROAST

Serv.: 2| **Prep.:** 15m | **Cook:** 30m

Ingredients:
- ✓ 1 eggplant, peeled and sliced
- ✓ 1 small head cauliflower, chopped
- ✓ 1/4 cup olive oil
- ✓ 1 teaspoon curry powder
- ✓ 1 teaspoon ground cumin
- ✓ 1/2 teaspoon garlic salt
- ✓ 6 fresh basil leaves, sliced

Directions: Set the oven to 400°F (200°C) and start preheating. Line parchment paper on a baking sheet.

In a large bowl that comes with a lid, place cauliflower and eggplant.

In a separate bowl, whisk together basil, garlic salt, ground cumin, curry powder and olive oil; add to cauliflower and eggplant mixture. Cover with the lid and shake until vegetables are well coated.

Place cauliflower and eggplant on prepared baking sheet.

Bake in preheated oven for about 30 minutes until caramelized and brown in color.

CAULIFLOWER RADISH GARLIC MASH

Serv.: 8| **Prep.:** 20m | **Cook:** 10m

Ingredients:
- ✓ 4 cloves garlic, roughly chopped, or more to taste
- ✓ 2 heads cauliflower, roughly chopped
- ✓ 2 cups roughly chopped radishes
- ✓ Freshly ground black pepper to taste
- ✓ 1 pinch salt to taste (optional)

Directions: Mix together garlic and water then boil in a big pot. Add radishes and cauliflower; mix and cook for 5-10 minutes till cauliflower is pierced with fork easily and tender. Strain; keep cooking liquid. Transfer flower mixture into a bowl.

Blend cauliflower mixture with a handheld mixer till smooth; thin with some cooking liquid. Season using salt and pepper.

CAULIFLOWER RICE

Serv.: 4| **Prep.:** 10m | **Cook:** 10m

Ingredients:
- ✓ 1 head cauliflower, broken into florets
- ✓ 3 tablespoons butter
- ✓ 1 clove garlic, minced, or to taste
- ✓ 1/2 teaspoon cumin
- ✓ 1/2 teaspoon ground coriander
- ✓ 1/2 teaspoon garam masala
- ✓ 1/2 teaspoon ground turmeric
- ✓ 1/4 teaspoon minced fresh ginger, or to taste
- ✓ 1 pinch cayenne pepper, or more to taste
- ✓ Salt and ground black pepper to taste
- ✓ 1 lime, cut into wedges
- ✓ 1/4 cup chopped fresh cilantro, or to taste

Directions: In a food processor or blender, pulse

the cauliflower florets until broken into rice-sized pieces.

On medium-high heat, heat butter in a frying pan; add black pepper, cauliflower rice, salt, garlic, cayenne pepper, cumin, ginger, coriander, turmeric, and garam masala. Cook for 10m while mixing from time to time until the cauliflower is soft.

Take off heat then top with cilantro and lime wedges.

CEDAR PLANK GRILLED SALMON WITH GARLIC & LEMON

Serv.: 8 | **Prep.:** 15m | **Cook:** 20m

Ingredients:
- ✓ 1 (3 pound) whole filet of salmon
- ✓ 6 tablespoons extra-virgin olive oil
- ✓ 4 large garlic cloves, minced
- ✓ 1/4 cup minced fresh dill
- ✓ 2 teaspoons salt
- ✓ 1 teaspoon ground black pepper
- ✓ 1 teaspoon lemon zest, plus lemon wedges for serving

Directions: Select a large, untreated cedar plank (or planks) enough to hold a side of salmon, about 16 to 20 inches in length and 5 to 7 inches in width. Soak plank in water for 30 minutes up to 24 hours. Put something heavy on top to keep the plank submerged (like a brick).

Prepare the grill. Turn grill burners on high for about 10 minutes. If using a coal grill, build a charcoal fire on half the grill. Meanwhile, combine garlic, dill, lemon zest, oil, salt and pepper. Spread mixture over salmon, coating even into the scored areas.

Take the soaked cedar and place on the hot grill grate. Cover and keep it closed for 5 minutes, watch until wood starts to smoke. Arrange salmon in the hot plank and move it away from direct charcoal heat or turn burners down to low. Keep covered and cook for 20 to 25 minutes or until salmon has turned transparent throughout. Grilling time might take longer depending on the grill temperature and thickness. To confirm if fish is done, insert a thermometer in the thickest section

of the fish, it should read 130 degrees. Let it stand for 5 minutes then serve with lemon slices.

MUSTARD

Serv.: 64 | **Prep.:** 15m | **Cook:** 25m

Ingredients:
- ✓ 1 1/2 cups white wine
- ✓ 1 cup water, or more as needed
- ✓ 2/3 cup white wine vinegar
- ✓ 1 yellow onion, chopped
- ✓ 2 cloves garlic, minced
- ✓ 1 cup whole yellow mustard seeds
- ✓ 1/4 cup dry mustard
- ✓ 1 tablespoon garlic powder
- ✓ 1 teaspoon salt
- ✓ 4 1-pint canning jars with lids and rings

Directions: In a saucepan, mix garlic with onion, vinegar, water and white wine; boil, lower the heat to medium low, then simmer for 15 minutes, until flavors blend. Cool to room temperature then pour into a big bowl through a strainer; save the liquid then remove garlic and onions.

Into the strained liquid, mix the salt, garlic powder, dry mustard and mustard seeds; cover the bowl using plastic wrap then allow to sit at room temperature for 24 to 48 hours, until the mixture thickens.

Puree the mustard mixture with a stick blender to achieve the desired texture. Move the mustard mixture to a saucepan then put in water if necessary to achieve a smooth texture. Simmer the mustard, lower the heat to medium, then cook for 10 minutes, mixing constantly, until flavors blend together.

Pack the mustard into hot, sterilized jars then fill up to 1/4 inch of the top. Run a thin spatula or knife around the jars ' inside after filling them to avoid any air bubbles. To discard any food residue, clean the jars' rims by wiping with a damp paper towel. Add the lids on top then screw on the rings.

Refrigerate the mustard for a minimum of 1 week, until the flavors combine.

FRIED SWEET PLANTAINS

Serv.: 4| **Prep.:** 5m | **Cook:** 15m

Ingredients:
- ✓ 1/4 cup vegetable oil
- ✓ 2 very ripe plantains (about 3/4 pound each), peeled and cut on the diagonal into 1/2-inch slices
- ✓ Salt to taste
- ✓ 1 lime, cut in wedges (optional)

Directions: In a heavy-duty skillet, heat oil on high heat. Put into the pan with 4-5 plantain slices, arrange in one layer and cook for 4-6 minutes on each side, until softened and golden brown. Turn out onto a plate lined with paper towel, then repeat the process with the rest of plantain slices. Sprinkle with salt and drizzle with lime over the cooked plantains.

HARISSA SAUCE

Serv.: 6| **Prep.:** 20m | **Cook:** 15m

Ingredients:
- ✓ 2 red bell peppers, halved and seeded
- ✓ 6 Fresno chile peppers
- ✓ 1 habanero pepper
- ✓ 2 tablespoons vegetable oil
- ✓ 1/4 teaspoon caraway seeds, or more to taste
- ✓ 1/4 teaspoon coriander seeds, or more to taste
- ✓ 1/2 teaspoon ground cumin
- ✓ 1/2 teaspoon dried mint
- ✓ 1 teaspoon kosher salt, or to taste
- ✓ 4 garlic cloves, peeled
- ✓ 1 lemon, juiced
- ✓ 1 tablespoon extra-virgin olive oil

Directions: Place oven rack approximately 6 inches far from the source of heat and preheat the oven's broiler. Use aluminum foil to line a baking sheet. On the prepared baking sheet, place red bell peppers, cut-side down. Cook under the preheated broiler for 5-8 minutes, until the skins of peppers has blistered and blackened. Put the blackened peppers into a bowl and use plastic wrap to seal tightly. Allow the peppers to steam as they cool for 20 minutes. Get rid of the skins.

Bring lightly salted water in a big pot to a boil. Put in habanero and Fresno Chiles and cook on moderate heat, without a cover, for 3 minutes, until vegetables begin to soften. Drain and set aside to allow the vegetables to cool. Get rid of membranes and seeds from the Chiles (remember to wear gloves), then set aside.

In a skillet, shake together caraway seeds and coriander on moderate heat for 2 minutes, until you begin to smell the spice. Crush toasted seeds with a mortar and pestle, then put in salt, mint and cumin, crush until ground finely. Turn spices to a blender and put in vegetable oil, lemon juice, garlic, Chiles and roasted bell peppers. Puree until smooth, then pour in extra-virgin olive oil at the end. Blend just several seconds.

CHICKEN THIGHS WITH TURMERIC AND SEA SALT

Serv.: 2| **Prep.:** 10m | **Cook:** 16m

Ingredients:
- ✓ 1 (1 inch) piece turmeric root, peeled and diced
- ✓ 1/2 teaspoon sea salt
- ✓ 2 boneless, skinless chicken thighs
- ✓ 1 1/2 teaspoons vegetable oil

Directions: Use a mortar and pestle to grind sea salt and turmeric into a fine paste. Rub chicken thighs evenly with the paste. Cover with plastic wrap and put to one side for about 1 hour to allow flavors to develop. In a large skillet, heat oil over medium heat. Cook chicken in hot oil for about 8 minutes until underside turns brown. Turn over and cook the other side for about 8 more minutes until browned. An inserted instant-read thermometer into the chicken should reach165°F (74°C)

CHICKEN AND PEPPERS EGG DROP STEW

Serv.: 2| **Prep.:** 30m | **Cook:** 18m

Ingredients:

- ✓ 1 tablespoon olive oil
- ✓ 1 (8 ounce) boneless chicken breast, cut into bite-size pieces
- ✓ 2 links hot chicken sausage, cut into 1-inch slices
- ✓ 1 yellow onion, sliced
- ✓ 1 red bell pepper, thinly sliced
- ✓ 1 poblano pepper, sliced
- ✓ 1 jalapeno pepper, seeded and thinly sliced
- ✓ 1 teaspoon sea salt
- ✓ 1/2 teaspoon freshly ground black pepper
- ✓ 4 cups low-sodium chicken broth
- ✓ 1 tablespoon unsalted butter
- ✓ 1 tablespoon arrowroot powder
- ✓ 2 eggs
- ✓ 2 tablespoons chopped fresh parsley, or more to taste

Directions: Use a big pot and heat oil on medium high heat. Add in the sausage and chicken. Stir and cook for about 7 minutes until evenly brown. Mix in the red bell pepper, onion, jalapeno pepper, poblano pepper, black pepper and salt. Cook for another 5 to 7 minutes until soft, frequently stir. Transfer the chicken broth to the pot and let it boil. Lower the heat to medium heat; then stir in the arrowroot powder and butter.
Whisk eggs in a separate mixing bowl.
Adjust the heat to medium high and bring the mixture to an active simmer. Take off heat then put in the eggs slowly while stirring using a wooden spoon for about a minute. Add in parsley.

Chicken and Peppers with Balsamic Vinegar

Serv.: 4| **Prep.:** 15m | **Cook:** 40m

Ingredients:

- ✓ 1/4 cup olive oil, divided
- ✓ 4 skinless, boneless chicken breast halves - cut into strips
- ✓ Salt and pepper to taste
- ✓ 1 red bell pepper, thinly sliced
- ✓ 1 yellow bell pepper, thinly sliced
- ✓ 1 orange bell pepper, thinly sliced
- ✓ 1 medium onion, thinly sliced
- ✓ 4 large cloves garlic, finely chopped
- ✓ 1 tablespoon dried basil
- ✓ 1/4 cup balsamic vinegar, divided

Directions: In a large skillet, bring 2 tablespoons of olive oil to medium-high heat. Bring chicken into the skillet, add pepper and salt to season and brown each side. Turn off the heat and put aside. In the skillet, bring the rest of the oil to medium heat, then mix in onion, orange bell pepper, yellow bell pepper and red bell pepper. Cook until softened, about 5 minutes. Stir in garlic; cook, stirring, for about 60 seconds. Blend in 2 tablespoons of balsamic vinegar and basil. Put chicken back into the skillet. Switch to low heat; simmer, covered, for 20 minutes until the juices run clear and no pink meat remains. Whisk in the rest of balsamic vinegar just before eating.

Chicken with Garlic, Basil, and Parsley

Serv.: 4| **Prep.:** 10m | **Cook:** 40m

Ingredients:

- ✓ 1 tablespoon dried parsley, divided
- ✓ 1 tablespoon dried basil, divided
- ✓ 4 skinless, boneless chicken breast halves
- ✓ 4 cloves garlic, thinly sliced
- ✓ 1/2 teaspoon salt
- ✓ 1/2 teaspoon crushed red pepper flakes
- ✓ 2 tomatoes, sliced

Directions: Set the oven to 175°C or 350°F to preheat. Use cooking spray to coat a 13"x9" baking dish.
Sprinkle evenly on the bottom of the baking dish with 1 tsp. of basil and 1 tsp. of parsley. Arrange in the dish with chicken breast halves, then sprinkle with garlic slices evenly. Combine together red pepper, salt, leftover 2 tsp. of basil, leftover 2 tsp. of parsley in a small bowl, then sprinkle over chicken. Put slices of tomato on top.
In the preheated oven, bake for about 25 minutes. Take off the cover and keep on baking until juices run clear, for 15 minutes.

CHILE PORK

Serv.: 10| **Prep.:** 10m | **Cook:** 2h

Ingredients:
- ✓ 2 tablespoons chili powder
- ✓ 1 teaspoon salt
- ✓ 2 1/2 teaspoons ground cumin
- ✓ 2 teaspoons minced garlic
- ✓ 1 tablespoon fresh cilantro
- ✓ 2 pounds pork tenderloin, cubed
- ✓ 1 dash ground black pepper

Directions: Combine pepper, garlic cilantro, cumin, salt, and chili powder together. Coat the pork cubes with the mixture and allow to sit in the fridge 45 minutes. Set an oven to 107°C (225°F) and start preheating. Bake until crispy, 2 hours.

CHILI POWDER

Serv.: 6| **Prep.:** 5m | **Cook:** 0

Ingredients:
- ✓ 2 tablespoons paprika
- ✓ 2 teaspoons oregano
- ✓ 1 1/2 teaspoons cumin
- ✓ 1 1/2 teaspoons garlic powder
- ✓ 3/4 teaspoon onion powder
- ✓ 1/2 teaspoon cayenne pepper

Directions: In a bowl, mix together cayenne pepper, onion powder, garlic powder, cumin, oregano and paprika.

CHILI LIME CHICKEN KABOBS

Serv.: 4| **Prep.:** 15m | **Cook:** 15m

Ingredients:
- ✓ 3 tablespoons olive oil
- ✓ 1 1/2 tablespoons red wine vinegar
- ✓ 1 lime, juiced
- ✓ 1 teaspoon chili powder
- ✓ 1/2 teaspoon paprika
- ✓ 1/2 teaspoon onion powder
- ✓ 1/2 teaspoon garlic powder
- ✓ Cayenne pepper to taste
- ✓ Salt and freshly ground black pepper to taste
- ✓ 1 pound skinless, boneless chicken breast halves - cut into 1 1/2 inch pieces
- ✓ Skewers

Directions: Whisk lime juice, olive oil, and vinegar in a small bowl. Sprinkle with salt, black pepper, paprika, chili powder, garlic powder, onion powder, and cayenne pepper. In a shallow baking dish, put the chicken and pour the sauce, stirring to coat the chicken. Put on the lid and refrigerate for at least an hour.
Preheat grill on medium-high. Skewer chicken. Dispose of the marinade.
Lightly great the grates. Grill chicken until juices run clear, about 10 to 15 minutes.

CHILI ROASTED KALE

Serv.: 4| **Prep.:** 15m | **Cook:** 10m

Ingredients:
- ✓ 4 cups kale, washed and stems removed
- ✓ 1 tablespoon extra-virgin olive oil
- ✓ 1 tablespoon chili powder
- ✓ 1/2 teaspoon kosher salt

Directions: Set the oven to 200°C or 400°F to preheat.
In a big mixing bowl, add the kale and use olive oil to drizzle over. Toss together until coated evenly, then sprinkle kosher salt and chili powder over and toss together one more time. Spread onto a baking sheet with the seasoned kale.
In the preheated oven, roast about 5 minutes, then stir in kale and keep on roasting for 5-8 minutes, until the edges are slightly crispy and brown. Serve instantly.

CHILLED VEGETABLE SALAD

Serv.: 6| **Prep.:** 25m | **Cook:** 0

Ingredients:
- ✓ 2 tomatoes, cut into chunks
- ✓ 1 large zucchini, cut into chunks

- ✓ 1 large yellow squash, cut into chunks
- ✓ 1/2 green bell pepper, diced
- ✓ 1/2 sweet red onion, chopped
- ✓ 2 cloves garlic, minced
- ✓ 1 teaspoon dried basil
- ✓ 1/2 teaspoon salt, or to taste
- ✓ 1/2 teaspoon ground black pepper, or to taste
- ✓ 1/4 cup olive oil
- ✓ 1/4 cup red wine vinegar
- ✓ 3 tablespoons water

Directions: Put black pepper, salt, basil, garlic, red onion, green bell pepper, yellow squash, zucchini and tomatoes in big bowl; add water, vinegar and olive oil. Toss to coat; refrigerate before serving for 1 hour.

CHINESE PICKLED CUCUMBERS

Serv.: 4| **Prep.:** 10m | **Cook:** 0

Ingredients:
- ✓ 1/2 teaspoon salt
- ✓ 1 large English cucumber, cut into 1/4 inch slices
- ✓ 3 tablespoons rice vinegar
- ✓ 3 tablespoons honey

Directions: In a colander in the sink, add cucumber slices and sprinkle lightly over with salt, then toss to coat well. Let the cucumber drain about a half hour. Shake the colander gently to get rid of any excess liquid and turn the cucumber to a big bowl. Stir in honey and rice vinegar, ensuring to coat each cucumber slice equally. Cover and chill overnight. Toss cucumber and turn it back to the fridge for an hour more. Serve chilled.

CHIPOTLE OIL

Serv.: 20| **Prep.:** 5m | **Cook:** 3m

Ingredients:
- ✓ 1 1/2 cups olive oil
- ✓ 1/2 cup dried chipotle chile pepper, crushed
- ✓ 1/2 cup red pepper flakes

Directions: In a saucepan, add oil on moderate

heat. Heat oil to 120°C or 250°F with a candy thermometer to measure temperature.

In a spice grinder, add small pieces of broken chipotle chiles and pulse to grind into 1/8" pieces. Stir into the hot oil with red pepper flakes and ground chipotle chiles. Cook for 3-5 minutes, until chile oil starts to foam.

Take chili oil away from the heat, then cover and allow to sit about 4 hours to overnight. Pour chile oil into a sealable container through a fine mesh strainer.

CHIPOTLE TACO BURGER

Serv.: 4| **Prep.:** 15m | **Cook:** 15m

Ingredients:
- ✓ 1 pound ground beef
- ✓ 1/4 cup diced onion
- ✓ 3 chipotle peppers in adobo sauce, seeded and diced
- ✓ 1 teaspoon taco seasoning

Directions: Preheat an outdoor grill to medium high heat; oil the grate lightly.

Thoroughly mix taco seasoning, chipotle peppers, onion and ground beef in a bowl using your hands; form to 4 patties.

On the preheated grill, cook burgers, 7-10 minutes per side, till grey in middle, hot and firm. An instant-read thermometer inserted in the middle should read 70°C/160°F.

CHOCOLATE, ALMOND COCONUT VEGAN FAT BOMBS

Serv.: 20| **Prep.:** 10m | **Cook:** 0

Ingredients:
- ✓ 1 cup shredded unsweetened coconut, divided
- ✓ 1/2 cup melted coconut oil
- ✓ 1/2 cup almonds, finely chopped
- ✓ 1/2 cup coconut milk
- ✓ 1/2 cup chopped Medjool dates
- ✓ 1 tablespoon low-calorie natural sweetener (such as Swerve®)

Directions: In the bowl of a food processor, blend sweetener, half cup of shredded coconut, coconut milk, coconut oil, dates, and almonds for about 2 minutes until the resulting mixture is creamy. Place in a freezer for about 15 minutes until set.

Form the mixture into one-inch balls and then roll into the remaining half cup of shredded coconut.

CHOP CHOP SALAD

Serv.: 6| **Prep.:** 20m | **Cook:** 0

Ingredients:
- ✓ 1 red grapefruit
- ✓ 1 cup peeled, chopped jicama
- ✓ 1 cup chopped orange bell pepper
- ✓ 1 cup chopped cucumber
- ✓ 1 tomato, chopped
- ✓ 2 green onions, chopped
- ✓ 1/4 cup chopped fresh cilantro

Directions: Cut a slice at the top and bottom of the grapefruit, slicing into the fruit, using a very sharp knife. Stand the grapefruit up on a work surface. Slice off the peel and white pith in vertical slices exposing the fruit segments, slightly cutting into fruit part. Gently slice between exposed white membranes with a knife. Loosen the grapefruit segments into a bowl. Take out any seeds.

Put cilantro, green onions, tomato, cucumber, orange bell pepper, jicama, and grapefruit sections in a salad boss. Gently toss to mix.

CHOPPED CHICKEN

Serv.: 8| **Prep.:** 15m | **Cook:** 30m

Ingredients:
- ✓ 2 tablespoons rendered chicken fat
- ✓ 2 onions, diced
- ✓ 1 pound chicken livers, rinsed
- ✓ 2 tablespoons rendered chicken fat
- ✓ 3 hard-cooked egg yolks
- ✓ 1 teaspoon salt
- ✓ 1/4 teaspoon freshly ground black pepper

Directions: Place a large skillet on the stove and turn on to medium-low heat then put in 2 tablespoons of chicken fat and stir in onions, regularly stir for about 20 minutes until brown in color. Place the onions to food processor, leave the fat in the skillet. Let the chicken livers cook in a hot skillet for about 10 minutes until softened, light in color, and color red in the middle faded.

Then add the livers into the food processor with onions and stir in black pepper, salt, egg yolks, and 2 tablespoons chicken fat. Blend for 1 to 2minutes until texture becomes smooth.

CHOPPED LIVER

Serv.: 24| **Prep.:** 15m | **Cook:** 45m

Ingredients:
- ✓ 4 eggs
- ✓ 1 1/2 pounds beef liver, rinsed
- ✓ 1 pound chicken livers, rinsed
- ✓ 2 tablespoons corn oil
- ✓ 2 tablespoons rendered chicken fat
- ✓ 2 tablespoons corn oil
- ✓ 4 cups chopped onion
- ✓ 2 teaspoons salt
- ✓ 1/2 teaspoon ground black pepper
- ✓ 1 tablespoon rendered chicken fat

Directions: Put the eggs into a saucepan in one layer and fill it in with water enough to cover the eggs by an inch. Cover the saucepan and allow the water to boil on high heat. Once it boils, take it off from heat and allow the eggs to sit under hot water for 15 minutes. Pour the hot water out, then cool the eggs in the sink under a cold running water. Peel the shells once cold.

Set the oven's broiler for preheating and place the oven rack 6 inches apart from the heat source. Coat the chicken livers and beef with 2 tablespoons of corn oil, and spread the livers on a baking sheet. Let it broil inside the preheated oven for 8-10 minutes until it becomes brown on the top. Turn the livers and continue broiling for roughly 5 minutes until the livers are doesn't appear pinkish in the middle and juices run clear. Put the livers in a bowl and keep inside the fridge to chill.

Pour 2 tablespoons corn oil and 2 tablespoons of chicken fat and heat in a big skillet over medium-high heat. Add in the onion; stir while it cooks for about 10 minutes until softened and turned translucent. Lower the heat to medium-low, and continue to cook and stir for 15 to 20 minutes more until the onion becomes very tender and dark brown. Put the onion in a bowl; keep in the fridge while covered until chilled.

Chop the chilled onions, chilled beef and chicken livers, and hardboiled eggs finely together, then place in a bowl. Add in the leftover 1 tablespoon of chicken fat and stir. Spice the mixture up with pepper and salt. Keep in the fridge until serving it in.

ALGERIAN POTATO STEW

Serv.: 4| **Prep.:** 10m | **Cook:** 45m

Ingredients:
Dersa:
- ✓ 4 cloves garlic, peeled and halved
- ✓ 1 small fresh red chile pepper, seeded and chopped
- ✓ 1 teaspoon ground cumin
- ✓ 1 teaspoon paprika
- ✓ 1/2 teaspoon black pepper
- ✓ 1/2 teaspoon cayenne pepper
- ✓ 1/2 teaspoon salt
- ✓ 2 tablespoons olive oil
Stew:
- ✓ 1 1/2 pounds new potatoes, halved
- ✓ 1 tablespoon tomato paste
- ✓ Water to cover
- ✓ Salt to taste

Directions: In a mortar, mix salt, cayenne, black pepper, paprika, cumin, chile pepper and garlic; grind with a pestle till a paste forms. Put in olive oil; combine dersa properly.

Place a large saucepan on medium heat; stir-fry the dersa for 2-4 minutes till fragrant. Put in potato halves; stir to incorporate with the dersa. Mix in tomato sauce. Transfer in enough water to just cover the potatoes; boil. Lower the heat; simmer for around 40 minutes, till the potatoes become tender.

Ladle the cooked potatoes into a serving bowl. Scoop any of the remaining sauce on top of the potatoes.

HOT SAUCE

Serv.: 16| **Prep.:** 10m | **Cook:** 0

Ingredients:
- ✓ 2 jalapeno peppers
- ✓ 1 (28 ounce) can whole tomatoes in juice
- ✓ 1 slice white onion
- ✓ 1 teaspoon minced garlic
- ✓ 1/2 teaspoon ground cumin
- ✓ 1/4 teaspoon dried oregano
- ✓ 1/4 teaspoon salt

Directions: Get rid of the stems from the jalapeno peppers, and the seeds from one jalapeno. In a blender, add salt, oregano, cumin, garlic, onion, tomatoes with liquid, and both jalapeno peppers, then process to wanted consistency and serve.

COCONUT MAPLE COFFEE

Serv.: 1| **Prep.:** 10m | **Cook:** 0

Ingredients:
- ✓ 2 tablespoons maple syrup
- ✓ 2 tablespoons unsweetened coconut milk
- ✓ 1 cup brewed coffee

Directions: In a large mug, combine coconut milk and maple syrup together. Stir in coffee.

COCONUT CRUSTED TARO FRIES

Serv.: 2| **Prep.:** 10m | **Cook:** 30m

Ingredients:
- ✓ 2 tablespoons coconut milk
- ✓ 1 tablespoon coconut oil, melted
- ✓ 1 pinch Himalayan salt
- ✓ 1 large taro root, peeled and sliced into thin strips
- ✓ 1 tablespoon coconut flakes

Directions: Preheat oven to 400°F (200°C).

In a bowl, mix salt, coconut oil, and coconut milk together. Add taro root. Toss to evenly coat. Arrange the coated taro root on a baking sheet. Sprinkle the taro root with coconut flakes. Use your hands to mix thoroughly.

Bake in the oven for 15 minutes. Flip and continue baking for another 15 minutes until coconut is golden and crispy.

Cod in Tomatoes with Wine

Serv.: 2| **Prep.:** 30m | **Cook:** 25m

Ingredients:
- ✓ 6 vine-ripened tomatoes
- ✓ 1 tablespoon vegetable oil
- ✓ 3/4 onion, finely chopped
- ✓ 2 cloves garlic, chopped
- ✓ 1 fresh red chile pepper, seeded and chopped
- ✓ 1 cup dry white wine, or more as needed
- ✓ Salt and ground black pepper to taste
- ✓ 1/4 cup chopped fresh basil
- ✓ 2 tablespoons chopped fresh parsley
- ✓ 2 (4 ounce) cod loins
- ✓ 8 large uncooked prawns, peeled and deveined

Directions: In the bottom of each tomato, cut an "X". Let a pot of water boil. Put in the tomatoes and let it cook in boiling water for 2 minutes. Use a slotted spoon to remove the tomatoes from the pot and put it in a bowl with iced water for 1 minute. Remove the skin of the tomatoes from the "X" side up then slice.

Heat vegetable oil in a skillet over low heat. Sauté garlic and onion for about 2 minutes until fragrant. Put in the tomatoes and chile pepper and let it cook. Stir for 5-8 minutes until the tomatoes has started to reduce. Add in the wine and let it cook for approximately 5 more minutes over medium heat until the wine has reduced a little bit. Mix in the basil, parsley, salt and black pepper.

Put the cod loins into the tomato mixture then cover the skillet and let it cook for 5 minutes. Flip the cod over on the other side and let it cook for 3-5 minutes until the fish is flaking apart easily using a fork. Mix in the prawns. Cover the skillet again and let it cook for 2-3 minutes until the prawns are opaque on the inside and bright pink in color on the outside. Put in black pepper and salt to taste.

Colorful Spinach and Prosciutto Side

Serv.: 4| **Prep.:** 5m | **Cook:** 15m

Ingredients:
- ✓ 2 tablespoons olive oil
- ✓ 1 (10 ounce) package frozen chopped spinach, thawed and squeezed dry
- ✓ 4 ounces thinly sliced prosciutto, chopped
- ✓ 1 (4 ounce) jar roasted red peppers, drained and chopped
- ✓ 1 (6.5 ounce) jar artichoke hearts, drained and sliced
- ✓ 1 tablespoon garlic powder

Directions: In a large skillet, heat oil over medium-low heat. Add artichoke hearts, red peppers, prosciutto, and spinach. Sprinkle with garlic powder to season. Sauté and mix until vegetables are thoroughly heated, about 15 minutes.

Conch Ceviche with Pineapple

Serv.: 8| **Prep.:** 15m | **Cook:** 0

Ingredients:
- ✓ 2 pounds fresh conch, removed from shell
- ✓ 1/2 fresh pineapple - peeled, cored and chopped
- ✓ 1/2 cup water
- ✓ 2 lemons, juiced
- ✓ 1 cup chopped fresh cilantro
- ✓ 1 medium onion, chopped
- ✓ 1 medium tomato, chopped (optional)
- ✓ Salt to taste

Directions: Trim and peel the conch, then cut into small cubes. Put in a big bowl together with salt, tomato, pineapple, onion, cilantro, lemon juice and water. Before serving, allow to stand at room temperature for an hour.

CORIANDER CHICKEN WITH MANGO SALSA

Serv.: 2| **Prep.:** 30m | **Cook:** 15m

Ingredients:
- ✓ 1 skinless, boneless chicken breast
- ✓ 1/2 teaspoon salt
- ✓ 1 teaspoon black pepper
- ✓ 1 tablespoon ground coriander seed
- ✓ 2 tablespoons extra virgin olive oil
- ✓ 1 mango - peeled, seeded, and chopped
- ✓ 1 orange, peeled and chopped
- ✓ 1/3 red onion, chopped
- ✓ 1 red chile pepper, seeded and chopped
- ✓ 1 tablespoon chopped fresh cilantro
- ✓ 1/2 teaspoon black pepper

Directions: Season chicken breast with a teaspoon black pepper and salt; let it stand for 10 minutes. Coat the chicken breasts evenly with ground coriander.

On medium heat, heat olive oil in a pan; add the chicken breast. Cook both sides of chicken until well-browned and the center is not pink anymore; take off from heat. Let the chicken cool down before cutting.

Combine half teaspoon black pepper, mango, fresh cilantro, orange, chile pepper, and onion together in a bowl. Spread salsa over the chopped chicken breast; serve.

CORIANDER AND CUMIN RUBBED PORK CHOPS

Serv.: 2| **Prep.:** 10m | **Cook:** 15m

Ingredients:
- ✓ 1/2 teaspoon salt
- ✓ 1 tablespoon ground cumin
- ✓ 1 tablespoon ground coriander
- ✓ 3 cloves garlic, minced
- ✓ 2 tablespoons olive oil, divided
- ✓ 2 boneless pork loin chops
- ✓ Ground black pepper to taste

Directions: Combine 1 tablespoon of olive oil, garlic, coriander, cumin, and salt together until a paste is formed. Season pork chops with pepper and salt; rub seasoning paste all over pork chops. Heat the remaining olive oil over medium heat in a skillet; cook pork chops in heated oil until the internal temperature achieves 145°F (63°C), about 5 minutes per side.

CORNELL CHICKEN

Serv.: 6| **Prep.:** 5m | **Cook:** 47m

Ingredients:
- ✓ 2 cups cider vinegar
- ✓ 1 cup vegetable oil
- ✓ 1 egg
- ✓ 3 tablespoons salt
- ✓ 1 tablespoon poultry seasoning
- ✓ 1/2 teaspoon ground black pepper
- ✓ 1 (3 to 3 1/2 pound) broiler-fryer chicken, cut in half

Directions: Mix in a blender egg, oil, poultry seasoning, black pepper and cider vinegar. Place on the cover and blend until it becomes smooth.

Place blended mixture in a plastic resealable bag. Halve the chicken and rub with marinade, get rid of excess air, then seal. Place in the refrigerator to marinate for a minimum of 4 hours up to overnight.

Take out the halved chicken from the sealed bag and place on a plate or baking sheet with paper towels. Use extra paper towels to dry the chicken. Keep the marinade mixture.

Let griller heat up to medium-high heat and lightly grease the grate with oil.

In the heated griller, allow chicken to grill for 2 minutes with the skin side down. Flip each side and rub with marinade mixture and grill not then place on indirect heat.

Continue grilling and brushing glaze on for 45 minutes until both sides become brown and cooked well. Insert an instant thermometer read in the biggest part of the thigh and it should say 180°F or 82°C.

CORNELL CHICKEN MARINADE

Serv.: 24| **Prep.:** 10m | **Cook:** 0

Ingredients:
- ✓ 1 egg
- ✓ 1 cup vegetable oil
- ✓ 2 cups cider vinegar
- ✓ 3 tablespoons salt
- ✓ 1 tablespoon poultry seasoning
- ✓ 1 teaspoon ground black pepper

Directions: Crack and whisk an egg in a medium bowl until beaten. Slowly whisk in the oil until it blends completely. Mix in ground black pepper, poultry seasoning, salt, and vinegar. Save some sauce aside for basting later on. Coat the chicken with the sauce in a shallow baking dish. Cover and marinate the chicken in the refrigerator for 24 hours.

DEVILED EGGS CHESAPEAKE

Serv.: 12| **Prep.:** 25m | **Cook:** 15m

Ingredients:
- ✓ 6 eggs
- ✓ 4 ounces cooked blue crab meat
- ✓ 2 teaspoons vegetable oil
- ✓ 1 1/2 teaspoons seafood seasoning (such as Old Bay®), or as needed
- ✓ 1 1/2 teaspoons dry mustard
- ✓ 1/2 cup water, or as needed

Directions: Cover the eggs with water in a saucepan. Let it boil and remove it from the heat once done. Let the eggs stay in hot water for 15 minutes. Remove the eggs from the water and let it cool under cold running water. Peel the eggs. Slice the egg in half lengthwise. In a bowl, mash the egg yolks using a fork. Stir in 1 1/2 tsp. of seafood seasoning, dry mustard, crab meat, and oil. Beat the mixture on low speed using an electric mixer until well-combined. Slowly pour in water to the egg yolk mixture and beat at higher speed slowly until the mixture is smooth.

Arrange the egg whites on a serving platter. Spread the yolk mixture into the egg whites and sprinkle seafood seasoning on its top.

DILL GAZPACHO

Serv.: 6| **Prep.:** 25m | **Cook:** 0

Ingredients:
- ✓ 6 medium ripe tomatoes, finely chopped
- ✓ 2 cucumbers, peeled and finely chopped
- ✓ 1 onion, finely chopped
- ✓ 1 green bell pepper, finely chopped
- ✓ Jalapeno pepper, seeded and minced
- ✓ 1 large lemon, juiced
- ✓ 1 tablespoon balsamic vinegar
- ✓ 2 teaspoons olive oil
- ✓ 1 teaspoon kosher salt
- ✓ 1/2 teaspoon ground black pepper
- ✓ 1/4 cup chopped fresh dill

Directions: Mix together the jalapeno pepper, bell pepper, onion, cucumber and tomatoes in a big bowl, then season it with pepper, salt, olive oil, balsamic vinegar and lemon juice.
Puree 1/2 of the mixture in a food processor or blender until it has a smooth consistency. Put it back into the bowl, mix in dill and stir well. Put cover and let it chill in the fridge for a minimum of one hour prior to serving.

DIVA CURRY BLEND

Serv.: 1| **Prep.:** 10m | **Cook:** 0

Ingredients:
- ✓ 1/4 cup ground coriander
- ✓ 1/4 cup ground cumin
- ✓ 1/4 cup ground turmeric
- ✓ 2 tablespoons ground cardamom
- ✓ 2 tablespoons yellow mustard seed
- ✓ 2 tablespoons ground ginger
- ✓ 2 tablespoons garlic powder
- ✓ 2 teaspoons cayenne pepper
- ✓ 1 teaspoon ground red chile pepper, or to taste
- ✓ 1/4 teaspoon ground cloves

Directions: In a bowl, combine together ground cloves, chili powder, cayenne pepper, garlic powder, ginger, mustard seed, cardamom, turmeric, cumin and coriander. Keep in a glass airtight container or jar.

KILLER SAUCE

Serv.: 8| **Prep.:** 25m | **Cook:** 1h

Ingredients:
- ✓ 1 pound lean ground beef
- ✓ 1 pound lean ground pork
- ✓ 1 onion, chopped, divided
- ✓ 4 cloves garlic, minced, divided
- ✓ 1 large green bell pepper, chopped
- ✓ 1 large red bell pepper, chopped
- ✓ 4 (29 ounce) cans tomato sauce
- ✓ 1 (4.5 ounce) can sliced mushrooms
- ✓ 1 tablespoon dried basil leaves, crushed
- ✓ 1 tablespoon dried oregano, crushed
- ✓ 2 tablespoons Italian seasoning
- ✓ 3 bay leaves
- ✓ 1 tablespoon red pepper flakes
- ✓ Salt to taste
- ✓ Ground black pepper to taste

Directions: Brown the onion, pork, and ground beef on medium heat in the big stockpot. Drain off the fat, and bring back to heat.
Whisk in tomato sauce, mushrooms, red and green pepper and garlic. Mix in the red pepper flakes, bay leaves, Italian seasoning, oregano and basil. Use the pepper and salt to taste.
Boil the sauce. Keep covered and lower the heat to low. Simmer for no less than 60 minutes or all day is better.

DRUNKEN FLAT IRON STEAK

Serv.: 6| **Prep.:** 5m | **Cook:** 10m

Ingredients:
- ✓ 1 (2 pound) flat iron steak
- ✓ 1/4 cup dry vermouth
- ✓ 1/4 cup sweet vermouth
- ✓ 2 1/2 tablespoons olive oil

- ✓ 1 tablespoon red pepper flakes

Directions: Put steak into a shallow dish or a large resealable bag. Pour in sweet vermouth and dry vermouth; stir properly to coat the steak. Cover or seal and let marinate for 6 hours in the refrigerator. Place a large skillet on medium heat; heat oil. Take the steak away from the bag; discard the marinade. Season red pepper flakes on both sides of the steak. Fry to your desired doneness, 3-4 minutes per side for medium-rare. Allow to rest for a few minutes before serving.

DRUNKEN FRUIT SALSA

Serv.: 6| **Prep.:** 15m | **Cook:** 1h

Ingredients:
- ✓ 1 medium mango, peeled and finely diced
- ✓ 3/4 cup chopped fresh strawberries
- ✓ 1 kiwi, peeled and finely diced
- ✓ 1 jalapeno pepper, seeded and finely chopped
- ✓ 2 tablespoons chopped fresh mint
- ✓ 1/4 cup rum

Directions: In a glass bowl, add and stir strawberries, mint, kiwi, mango, rum and jalapeno. Keep it refrigerated for 1-3 hours, stir once or twice.

EASIEST, AMAZING GUACAMOLE

Serv.: 8| **Prep.:** 5m | **Cook:** 0

Ingredients:
- ✓ 2 (6 ounce) avocados, pitted peeled and mashed
- ✓ 1/4 teaspoon coarse garlic salt

Directions: Mix well together the garlic salt and avocado in a bowl. Put one of avocado pits in to maintain the guacamole's freshness and preventing from turning brown.

EASY ALMOND THIN COOKIES

Serv.: 9| **Prep.:** 10m | **Cook:** 25m

Ingredients:
- ✓ 1 egg white, room temperature
- ✓ 1/3 cup coconut sugar
- ✓ 1/2 teaspoon almond extract
- ✓ 1/2 cup almond flour
- ✓ 1 tablespoon slivered almonds, chopped

Directions: Preheat an oven to 150 °C or 300 °F. Line parchment paper on a baking dish with, 8x8-inch in size.

In a bowl, beat almond extract, coconut sugar and egg white together. Into the egg mixture, fold the almond flour till barely blended; place the batter into the baking dish and spread out. Dust almonds over the batter and push down slightly.

In prepped oven, bake for 25 minutes till golden brown. To a cooling rack, put the cookies by lifting out parchment from baking dish. Allow to come to room temperature for an hour.

EASY CARAMELIZED ONION PORK CHOPS

Serv.: 4| **Prep.:** 5m | **Cook:** 40m

Ingredients:
- ✓ 1 tablespoon vegetable oil
- ✓ 4 (4 ounce) pork loin chops, 1/2 inch thick
- ✓ 3 teaspoons seasoning salt
- ✓ 2 teaspoons ground black pepper
- ✓ 1 onion, cut into strips
- ✓ 1 cup water

Directions: Rub the chops with 1 tsp. of the pepper and 2 tsp. of the seasoning salt or to taste.

In the skillet, heat the oil on medium heat. Brown the pork chops on each side. Put water and onions into pan. Keep covered, lower the heat, and let simmer for 20 minutes.

Flip the chops over, and put in leftover salt and pepper. Keep covered, and cook till the onions are light to medium brown and the water is evaporated. Take the chops out of the pan, and serve along with the onions over the top.

EASY CHICKEN TACO FILLING

Serv.: 4| **Prep.:** 10m | **Cook:** 20m

Ingredients:
- ✓ 2 skinless, boneless chicken breast halves
- ✓ 1/4 onion, sliced
- ✓ 1/4 green bell pepper, sliced

Directions: Sauté bell peppers and onion in a medium pan until they turn soft.

Place the chicken breasts atop the sautéed mixture and spray them with cooking spray.

Fry the chicken along with the sautéed mixture until brown and cooked through, shredding or cutting the chicken as it cooks.

EASY GARLIC GINGER CHICKEN

Serv.: 4| **Prep.:** 15m | **Cook:** 25m

Ingredients:
- ✓ 4 skinless, boneless chicken breast halves
- ✓ 3 cloves crushed garlic
- ✓ 3 tablespoons ground ginger
- ✓ 1 tablespoon olive oil
- ✓ 4 limes, juiced

Directions: Pound the chicken to 1/2-inch thickness. Combine lime juice, oil, ginger, and garlic in a large resealable plastic bag. Seal up the bag and shake until combined. Open the bag and put in the chicken. Seal it again and marinate in the fridge for no more than 20 minutes.

Take the chicken out of the bag; broil or grill, basting with the marinade, until the juices run clear and cooked through. Discard any leftover marinade.

EASY GARLIC KALE

Serv.: 4| **Prep.:** 10m | **Cook:** 10m

Ingredients:
- ✓ 1 bunch kale
- ✓ 1 tablespoon olive oil
- ✓ 1 teaspoon minced garlic

Directions: In a big bowl of water, steep kale leaves for 2 minutes, until sand and dirt start to fall to the bottom. Lift kale from the bowl without drying the leaves and get rid of the stems promptly. Chop kale leaves into pieces with 1 inch size.

In a big skillet, heat olive oil on moderate heat, then cook and stir garlic for 1 minute, until sizzling. Put into the skillet with kale and put a cover on top.

Cook for 5-7 minutes while stirring sometimes with tongs, until kale is lightly softened and bright green.

EASY GRILLED CHICKEN WINGS

Serv.: 20| **Prep.:** 10m | **Cook:** 30m

Ingredients:
- ✓ 20 chicken wings
- ✓ 2 tablespoons olive oil, or more as needed
- ✓ 3 teaspoons garlic salt
- ✓ 3 teaspoons ground black pepper

Directions: Set an outdoor grill to high heat to preheat and grease the grate lightly.

Tuck in the chicken wing flaps so that the wing will form a triangle.

In a large bowl, mix olive oil with some of the pepper and garlic salt. Put in a few chicken wings and flip to coat with the seasonings. Add more wings, the remaining pepper, and remaining garlic salt; flip to coat. Repeat the process until all wings are well-coated. Arrange on the preheated grill. Grill until the wings are softened, well browned, the juices run clear, and not anymore pink at the bone, for about 30-40 minutes; flip several times and rearrange them so they're evenly cooked.

EASY GUACAMOLE

Serv.: 16| **Prep.:** 10m | **Cook:** 0

Ingredients:
- ✓ 2 avocados
- ✓ 1 small onion, finely chopped
- ✓ 1 clove garlic, minced
- ✓ 1 ripe tomato, chopped

- ✓ 1 lime, juiced
- ✓ Salt and pepper to taste

Directions: Prepare a medium size serving bowl and put in the peeled avocados then crush it. Add in the pepper, salt, lime juice, tomato, garlic and onion the mix well. Add salt, pepper and left lime juice to taste. Let it chill for 1 hour to enhance the flavors.

EASY YET ROMANTIC FILET MIGNON

Serv.: 2| **Prep.:** 5m | **Cook:** 15m

Ingredients:
- ✓ 2 (8 ounce) (1 inch thick) filet mignon steaks
- ✓ 2 teaspoons olive oil
- ✓ 1/4 teaspoon onion powder
- ✓ Salt and pepper to taste
- ✓ 2 tablespoons minced shallot
- ✓ 2 slices bacon

Directions: Put the oven rack at the highest position. Turn the oven to broil setting.

Rub the steaks with olive oil until fully coated. Season with onion powder. Put pepper and salt to taste. Enclose each steak in one slice of bacon then secure the ends with a toothpick.

Put the seasoned steaks on a broiler pan and let it cook in the broiler for 5-7 minutes. Flip the steaks over on the other side and top it with shallots. Let it broil for 5-7 more minutes until your desired doneness is achieved.

EASY AND QUICK STRAWBERRY SUMMER SALAD

Serv.: 4| **Prep.:** 15m | **Cook:** 0

Ingredients:
- ✓ 1 tablespoon red wine vinegar
- ✓ 1/2 shallot, diced
- ✓ Salt and ground black pepper to taste
- ✓ 2 tablespoons extra-virgin olive oil
- ✓ 4 cups mixed greens
- ✓ 2 baby cucumbers, sliced
- ✓ 2 cups strawberries, hulled

✓ 1 pinch sea salt

Directions: In a bowl, stir shallot and red wine vinegar together; add black pepper and salt to taste. Whisk in olive oil in a stream into the mixture till a dressing is formed.

In a large bowl, toss cucumbers and mixed greens; top the mixture with dressing and toss till coated. Toss in strawberries slightly. Add sea salt to taste. Serve.

DELICE EGGS

Serv.: 2| **Prep.:** 5m | **Cook:** 10m

Ingredients:
✓ 1/4 cup vegetable oil
✓ 1 teaspoon garam masala
✓ 1 teaspoon ground turmeric
✓ 1 teaspoon ground coriander
✓ Salt to taste
✓ 1/2 cup finely chopped onion
✓ 3 green chile peppers, sliced
✓ 2 large eggs

Directions: Place skillet over medium heat and heat the oil. Add salt, coriander, turmeric, and garam masala. Stir green chile peppers and onions in the seasoned oil and cook for 5 minutes, or until onion is slightly tender.

Crack in the eggs and add salt to season. Stir and cook eggs for 5 minutes until scrambled.

EGG AND BROCCOLI SCRAMBLE

Serv.: 1| **Prep.:** 5m | **Cook:** 20m

Ingredients:
✓ 1/2 cup broccoli florets
✓ 1 large egg
✓ 1 tablespoon breast milk or formula

Directions: Boil or steam broccoli florets until fully tender. Drain if essential and puree or mash until reaching your desired consistency. Allow to cool, then put in a sealed container in the fridge until ready to use.

Whisk egg. Whisk in formula or breast milk and a quarter cup (60 mL) of broccoli puree until well blended.

Over medium heat, heat a pan. Put in broccoli mixture and egg, cook while stirring frequently, until eggs are scrambled and fully cooked through. Take away from heat, allow to cool, then chop into small pieces that your baby can eat.

EGGPLANT CAVIAR

Serv.: 6| **Prep.:** 5m | **Cook:** 20m

Ingredients:
✓ 1 large eggplant
✓ 1/3 cup chopped onion
✓ 3 tablespoons olive oil
✓ 2 tablespoons chopped fresh dill
✓ 2 teaspoons kosher salt
✓ 1 teaspoon freshly ground black pepper

Directions: Set an oven to preheat to broiler setting.

Thoroughly rinse the eggplant, then use fork to prick the skin in several places. Put it on a baking tray and let it broil for 8-10 minutes in the preheated oven, until it becomes soft. Flip over the eggplant and let it broil for another 8-10 minutes. Take it out of the oven and cut it in half.

Use spoon to scoop out the eggplant pulp and put it in a medium bowl. Combine pepper, salt, dill, olive oil and onion. Serve it cold or hot.

EGGPLANT MIXED GRILL

Serv.: 6| **Prep.:** 15m | **Cook:** 12m

Ingredients:
✓ 2 tablespoons olive oil
✓ 2 tablespoons chopped fresh parsley
✓ 2 tablespoons chopped fresh oregano
✓ 2 tablespoons chopped fresh basil
✓ 1 tablespoon balsamic vinegar
✓ 1 teaspoon kosher salt
✓ 1/2 teaspoon black pepper
✓ 6 cloves garlic, minced
✓ 1 red onion, cut into wedges
✓ 18 spears fresh asparagus, trimmed

- ✓ 12 crimini mushrooms, stems removed
- ✓ 1 (1 pound) eggplant, sliced into 1/4 inch rounds
- ✓ 1 red bell pepper, cut into wedges
- ✓ 1 yellow bell pepper, cut into wedges

Directions: Mix the garlic, pepper, kosher salt, vinegar, basil, oregano, parsley and olive oil in a big resealable plastic bag. Put yellow and red bell peppers, together with the eggplant, mushrooms, asparagus and onion into the bag; seal. Marinate it in the fridge, occasionally turning, for 2 hours. Preheat a grill to high heat.
Oil the grill grate lightly. Grill vegetables till tender, 6 minutes per side.

ROASTED VEGETABLE SALAD

Serv.: 10| **Prep.:** 20m | **Cook:** 35m

Ingredients:
- ✓ 1 eggplant - quartered lengthwise, and sliced into 1/2 inch pieces
- ✓ 2 small yellow squash, halved lengthwise and sliced
- ✓ 4 cloves garlic, peeled
- ✓ 1/4 cup olive oil, or as needed
- ✓ 1 red bell pepper, seeded and sliced into strips
- ✓ 1 bunch fresh asparagus, trimmed and cut into 2 inch pieces
- ✓ 1/2 red onion, sliced
- ✓ 1/4 cup red wine vinegar
- ✓ 2 tablespoons balsamic vinegar
- ✓ 1/4 cup olive oil
- ✓ 2 lemons, juiced
- ✓ 1/4 cup chopped fresh parsley
- ✓ 3 tablespoons chopped fresh oregano
- ✓ Salt and freshly ground black pepper to taste

Directions: Set an oven to 450°C (230°F). Grease a large baking sheet.
On the prepared baking sheet, evenly lay out eggplant and quash slices in layer. Place garlic cloves in one side of the pan so they can be found easily later. Bake in the preheated oven for 15 minutes.
While roasting the vegetables, put lemon juice, olive oil, balsamic vinegar and red wine vinegar together in a large serving bowl, whisk until well

combined. Add salt, pepper, parsley and oregano to season. Remove cloves of garlic from the oven and mash or chop into smaller pieces. Add garlic to dressing, whisk well and set aside.
Remove vegetables from the oven, and stir the eggplant and the squash well. Place asparagus, red onion and red bell pepper in layer on top of squash and eggplant. Put back in the oven and bake for an additional 15 to 20 minutes or until asparagus becomes soft but still has bright green color. Remove them from oven once vegetables are cooked well and slightly toasted. Place them in a bowl, pour in dressing, and stir until evenly coated. Taste and adjust the amount of salt and pepper if needed. Allow to chill for a few hours to marinate the vegetables.

PICKLED EGGS

Serv.: 12| **Prep.:** 30m | **Cook:** 5m

Ingredients:
- ✓ 12 eggs
- ✓ 1 cup white vinegar
- ✓ 1/2 cup water
- ✓ 2 tablespoons coarse salt
- ✓ 2 tablespoons pickling spice
- ✓ 1 onion, sliced
- ✓ 5 black peppercorns

Directions: In a big pot, put the eggs and cover in cold water. Boil water and immediately take off the heat. Place on the cover and allow the eggs to sit for 10 to 12 minutes in hot water. Take out of the hot water, let cool and remove shell. Into a wide mouth 1-quart jar, put the eggs.
Mix together black peppercorns, most of onion (set 2 slices aside), pickling spice, salt, water and vinegar in a saucepan. Let it come to a rolling boil; put on top of eggs in the jar. Top with 2 slices of onion and seal the jars. Let it come to room temperature, then chill for 3 days prior to serving.

ENERGIZING VEGAN MANGO BANANA CHIA SMOOTHIE

Serv.: 1| **Prep.:** 10m | **Cook:** 0

Ingredients:
- ✓ 1 mango, chopped, or more to taste
- ✓ 1 banana, sliced, or more to taste
- ✓ 3/4 cup cold water, or as needed
- ✓ 1/2 cup chopped romaine lettuce
- ✓ 2 ice cubes
- ✓ 1 teaspoon flax seeds (optional)
- ✓ 1 tablespoon chia seeds

Directions: Blend flax seeds, ice, lettuce, water, banana, and mango using a blender for about 2 minutes or until smooth. Add chia seeds to the mixture and stir. Let the smoothie sit for 2 minutes or until it thickens slightly.

ENERGY ELIXIR SMOOTHIE

Serv.: 1| **Prep.:** 10m | **Cook:** 0

Ingredients:
- ✓ 1 cup spring salad greens, or to taste
- ✓ 1 cup frozen red grapes
- ✓ 1 chopped frozen banana
- ✓ 1 cored and chopped frozen pear
- ✓ 2 tablespoons walnuts
- ✓ Water as needed

Directions: In a high-powered blender, put in walnuts, salad greens, pear, red grapes, and banana; pour in enough water to cover. Process it until smooth. Pour in more water until it reaches the preferred thickness.

EXOTIC SPICY EGGPLANT

Serv.: 6| **Prep.:** 30m | **Cook:** 25m

Ingredients:
- ✓ 2 tablespoons vegetable oil
- ✓ 1 (1 1/4 pound) eggplant, cut into 1-inch cubes
- ✓ 6 tablespoons vegetable oil
- ✓ 1/2 teaspoon cumin seeds
- ✓ 1/2 teaspoon fenugreek seeds, crushed
- ✓ 1/2 teaspoon kalonji (onion seed)
- ✓ 1/2 teaspoon sesame seeds
- ✓ 1 (1/2 inch) piece fresh ginger root, chopped
- ✓ 5 cloves garlic, chopped

- ✓ 2 onions, peeled and finely chopped
- ✓ 1 green chile pepper, seeded and chopped
- ✓ 1/4 cup tomato puree
- ✓ 1/2 teaspoon chili powder
- ✓ 1/2 teaspoon ground coriander
- ✓ 1/2 teaspoon ground turmeric
- ✓ 3/4 teaspoon salt
- ✓ 1/2 cup coconut milk
- ✓ 1 tablespoon cilantro leaves

Directions: Over medium-high heat, heat two tablespoons oil in large skillet and then fry pieces of eggplant for about 5 minutes until golden. Take out eggplant from skillet and put aside. Then use a paper towel to wipe out the skillet.

Over medium heat, heat six tablespoons of oil in the same skillet and then mix in sesame seeds, kalonji, fenugreek and cumin. Let it cook for about 2 minutes until cumin becomes golden. Lower the heat and then mix in garlic and ginger. Cook for several seconds. Mix in green chile pepper and onions. Continue cooking while stirring for about 10 minutes until onion is golden.

Mix salt, turmeric, coriander, chili powder and tomato puree into the onions. Cook while stirring for 2 minutes on medium heat or until oil separates. Mix in cooked eggplant. Cover the skillet and let it simmer for about 5 minutes until the eggplant is tender. Stir in coconut milk until heated through and blended. Drizzle with cilantro leaves.

EXTRA VIRGIN OLIVE OIL DIPPING SAUCE

Serv.: 4| **Prep.:** 5m | **Cook:** 0

Ingredients:
- ✓ 1/2 cup extra-virgin olive oil
- ✓ 1/2 teaspoon pressed garlic
- ✓ 1/2 teaspoon red pepper flakes
- ✓ 1/2 teaspoon dried parsley
- ✓ 1/2 teaspoon dried oregano
- ✓ 1/4 teaspoon kosher salt
- ✓ 1/4 teaspoon ground black pepper

Directions: In a small bowl, combine black pepper, kosher salt, oregano, parsley, red pepper flakes, garlic, and olive oil. Let marinate for 30 minutes at room temperature.

PRUNES & BACON

Serv.: 8| **Prep.:** 5m | **Cook:** 12m

Ingredients:
- ✓ 24 pitted prunes
- ✓ 12 bacon strips, cut in half
- ✓ 8 bamboo skewers, soaked in water for 20 minutes

Directions: Preheat oven to 175°C or 350°F.
Envelop each prune with bacon. Lace 3 bacon-wrapped prunes in a skewer. Place the skewers on a baking pan.
Bake in 350°F or 175°C oven for 12 minutes until the bacon is crisp; cool. Serve.

FABULOUS SPINACH SALAD

Serv.: 4| **Prep.:** 10m | **Cook:** 15m

Ingredients:
- ✓ 1 bunch fresh spinach - torn, washed and dried
- ✓ 10 fresh mushrooms, sliced
- ✓ 1 onion, thinly sliced
- ✓ 4 eggs
- ✓ 4 tomatoes, chopped
- ✓ Sea salt to taste
- ✓ 1/3 cup olive oil
- ✓ 1/8 cup rice wine vinegar

Directions: Add the eggs into a saucepan and use cold water to cover. Let the water boil. Put on the lid, take off the heat and leave the eggs in hot water for 10-12 minutes. Take out of the hot water, cool then peel and chop them.
Toss tomatoes, eggs, onion, mushrooms and spinach together and add salt for seasoning.
Mix the vinegar and oil together. Add to the salad and toss again to get them coated.

FALL HASH

Serv.: 5| **Prep.:** 15m | **Cook:** 35m

Ingredients:
- ✓ 1 pound Brussels sprouts
- ✓ 1 Pink Lady apple - peeled, cored and diced
- ✓ 2 tablespoons olive oil
- ✓ 1/4 teaspoon salt
- ✓ 3 ounces diced pancetta
- ✓ 1/4 cup thinly sliced red onion
- ✓ 1 clove garlic, chopped
- ✓ 1/2 head radicchio, outer leaves and core removed, quartered
- ✓ 1 tablespoon apple cider vinegar
- ✓ 1 tablespoon honey
- ✓ Reynolds Wrap® Aluminum Foil

Directions: Preheat the oven to 475°F. Start by getting rid of the leaves on the outer layer of Brussels sprouts and trimming the ends off. Using a food processor fitted with a slicing blade or a knife, cut into thin slices. Combine salt, olive oil, diced apples and the sprouts together by tossing. Use Reynolds Wrap® Aluminium Foil to line a sheet pan. Roast sprouts and apples for 20 minutes. Stir once midway through the process. Insert pancetta into a skillet, cooking at moderate heat for around 5 minutes until it turns crispy. Move the pancetta out of skillet, leaving 3 tablespoons of grease in there. Insert the garlic and onion, cooking for around 2 minutes. Insert radicchio and keep the quarters separate, stirring until the leaves are wilted. Insert the pancetta and Brussels sprouts, tossing until combined. Finish off by adding the honey and vinegar.

FAR EAST SPICED OLIVE OIL

Serv.: 16| **Prep.:** 5m | **Cook:** 0

Ingredients:
- ✓ 2 cups olive oil
- ✓ 2 whole star anise pods
- ✓ 3 whole cardamom pods
- ✓ 2 whole cloves

Directions: Mix cloves, cardamom, star anise and oil in a medium-sized glass mixing bowl. Whisk together and add mixture into the bottles, using a funnel. Keep it tightly covered and stored at room temperature.

FAST AND EASY SPINACH WITH SHALLOTS

Serv.: 4 | **Prep.:** 5m | **Cook:** 8m

Ingredients:
- ✓ 1 tablespoon olive oil
- ✓ 1 shallot, diced
- ✓ 1 (10 ounce) bag baby spinach leaves
- ✓ Kosher salt and freshly ground pepper to taste

Directions: Heat olive oil in a big skillet on moderate heat. Stir in shallots and cook about 5 minutes, until transparent. Put in spinach and sprinkle over with pepper and salt. Cook and stir for 3-5 minutes, until leaves are reduced and wilted.

FAST AND SIMPLE SALSA

Serv.: 28 | **Prep.:** 15m | **Cook:** 0

Ingredients:
- ✓ 6 large tomatoes, chopped
- ✓ 1 onion, chopped
- ✓ 3/4 cup green chile peppers, chopped
- ✓ 1 teaspoon vinegar
- ✓ 1 teaspoon salt

Directions: In a bowl, mix together green chile peppers, onion and tomatoes then drain quickly. Bring the mixture back to the bowl then stir into the tomato mixture with salt and vinegar.

FAT FREE BALSAMIC MARINADE

Serv.: 4 | **Prep.:** 5m | **Cook:** 0

Ingredients:
- ✓ 1/4 cup balsamic vinegar
- ✓ 1/4 cup white vinegar
- ✓ 1/4 cup water
- ✓ 1 tablespoon garlic powder
- ✓ 1 tablespoon onion powder
- ✓ 1/2 teaspoon salt
- ✓ 1/4 teaspoon dried thyme
- ✓ 1/4 teaspoon ground black pepper

Directions: In a bowl, whisk together pepper, thyme, salt, onion powder, garlic powder, water, white vinegar, and balsamic vinegar.

FAUX BOMBAY POTATOES

Serv.: 4 | **Prep.:** 5m | **Cook:** 20m

Ingredients:
- ✓ 3 turnips, diced
- ✓ 1/4 cup vegetable oil
- ✓ 1/2 teaspoon yellow mustard seed
- ✓ 1/2 teaspoon black mustard seed
- ✓ 1 1/2 teaspoons ground red pepper
- ✓ 1 teaspoon ground turmeric
- ✓ Salt to taste

Directions: Pour salted water over turnips to cover in a large pot. Bring to a boil over high heat, then turn heat to medium-low; simmer, covered for 15 to 20 minutes until tender. Drain off water and allow turnips to steam dry for 1 or 2 minutes. In a large skillet, heat oil over medium-high heat. Sauté turmeric, black mustard seeds, and yellow mustard seeds in hot oil until mustard seeds start to pop. Add turnips to the skillet. Cook, stirring for about 5 minutes until turnips is thoroughly heated. Sprinkle with salt to taste, and serve.

GRILLED CHICKEN BREAST WITH CUCUMBER & PEPPER RELISH

Serv.: 4 | **Prep.:** 15m | **Cook:** 15m

Ingredients:
- ✓ 1 cucumber - peeled, seeded and chopped
- ✓ 1 tablespoon chopped fresh parsley
- ✓ 1/8 cup chopped red onion
- ✓ 1/2 cup chopped yellow bell pepper
- ✓ 1/4 teaspoon crushed red pepper flakes
- ✓ 1/2 teaspoon ground cumin
- ✓ 1/8 teaspoon chili powder
- ✓ 2 tablespoons olive oil

- ✓ 4 skinless, boneless chicken breasts

Directions: For relish: combine red pepper flakes, bell pepper, chopped onion, parsley and cucumber in a medium bowl. Put aside.
Blend chili powder and cumin with olive oil in a small bowl. Rub chicken with the mixture, then bring into a shallow dish. Leave in the fridge to marinate for at least 60 minutes.
Start preheating the grill to medium heat.
Grease grill grate with a thin layer of oil. Grill chicken until the juices run clear, 8 minutes on each side. Serve with cucumber relish.

GRILLED CHICKEN WITH FRESH MANGO SALSA

Serv.: 4 | **Prep.:** 15m | **Cook:** 25m

Ingredients:
- ✓ 4 boneless, skinless chicken breast halves
- ✓ Salt and freshly ground black pepper to taste
- ✓ 1 tablespoon olive oil
- ✓ 2 cloves garlic, peeled and minced
- ✓ 1 (1/2 inch) piece fresh ginger root, minced
- ✓ 2 mangos - peeled, seeded, and diced
- ✓ 2 tablespoons cider vinegar
- ✓ 1 teaspoon white wine
- ✓ 1/4 cup chopped fresh cilantro

Directions: Preheat an outdoor grill for high heat; lightly coat a grate with oil.
Rub pepper and salt on chicken breast halves. Arrange on the prepared grill. Cook till the juices run clear and the meat is not pink anymore, 10-15 minutes per side. Take away from the heat; set aside and keep warm.
Place a medium skillet with oil on medium heat; sauté in garlic for around 1 minute. Stir in mangos and ginger; cook till the mangos turn tender, 3-4 minutes. Transfer in white wine and cider vinegar. Season with pepper and salt. Mix in cilantro; take away from the heat. Transfer on top of the grilled chicken. Serve.

GRILLED CIPOLLINI ONIONS

Serv.: 4 | **Prep.:** 15m | **Cook:** 10m

Ingredients:
- ✓ 2 wooden skewers, or as needed
- ✓ 12 cipollini onions, peeled
- ✓ 1/2 cup coarsely chopped fresh basil
- ✓ 1 tablespoon olive oil
- ✓ 1 teaspoon seasoned salt (such as LAWRY'S®)

Directions: Use water to fill shallow dish. In water, soak wooden skewers for 30 minutes.
In a bowl, toss salt, oil, basil and onions to coat onions. Refrigerate for 30-60 minutes till flavors merge.
Preheat outdoor grill to medium high heat; oil grate lightly.
On prepped skewers, thread onions, weaving the basil between the onions.
On preheated grill, cook onions, flip once, for 10 minutes or till tender and sweet.

GRILLED FLANK STEAK "PASTRAMI"

Serv.: 4 | **Prep.:** 10m | **Cook:** 16m

Ingredients:
- ✓ 1 tablespoon freshly ground black pepper
- ✓ 1 tablespoon ground coriander
- ✓ 1 tablespoon kosher salt
- ✓ 1 teaspoon paprika
- ✓ 1/2 teaspoon dry mustard
- ✓ 2 teaspoons vegetable oil
- ✓ 1 (1 1/2-pound) trimmed beef flank steak

Directions: In a bowl, combine dry mustard, paprika, kosher salt, coriander, and ground black pepper to make the rub.
Drizzle and evenly rub some vegetable oil on both sides of the flank steak. Poke holes on surface of both sides with a fork to let the meat absorb flavors more deeply. Rub thoroughly half of the spice mixture on each side and make sure to spread over surface equally. Wrap the steak using butcher paper and let it rest in the refrigerator for

2 hours to overnight. Before grilling, let the steak rest at room temperature for 30 minutes.

Preheat outdoor grill for medium-high heat and spread a thin layer of oil on the grate.

Grill for 8 minutes per side until steak is cooked to medium doneness, or until it reaches an internal temperature of 135 degrees F (57 degrees C). Remove from the grill and let it rest for a minimum of 5 minutes up to 15 minutes, until the temperature rises to 140 degrees F (60 degrees C) and juices are redistributed. Thinly slice against the grain and serve.

Grilled Fruit Kabobs

Serv.: 6| **Prep.:** 15m | **Cook:** 20m

Ingredients:
- ✓ 1/2 cup margarine
- ✓ 1/4 cup honey
- ✓ 3 fresh peaches, pitted and quartered
- ✓ 3 fresh plums, pitted and quartered
- ✓ 3 bananas, cut into 4 pieces each
- ✓ 12 strawberries, hulled
- ✓ 12 skewers

Directions: Preheat outdoor grill on medium. Secure a large foil sheet onto the grate.

Stir together honey and margarine in a small saucepan over medium heat until margarine melts. Reduce to low and cook with occasional stirring until thickened, about 5 minutes. Do not let boil. Skewer a strawberry, a quarter piece each of plum and peach, and a piece of banana. Place skewers on the foil in the grill and drizzle a spoonful of the honey-margarine mixture on each skewer.

Cook for about 5 minutes, or until fruit has softened and the sauce has thickened onto the fruit. Flip, drizzle another spoonful of the mixture, and grill for another 5 minutes.

Grilled Globe Squash

Serv.: 4| **Prep.:** 10m | **Cook:** 10m

Ingredients:
- ✓ 1/4 cup extra-virgin olive oil
- ✓ 2 tablespoons white vinegar
- ✓ 1/8 teaspoon salt
- ✓ 1/8 teaspoon ground black pepper
- ✓ 4 baseball-size globe squash, cut into 1/2-inch thick slices

Directions: In a big bowl, mix black pepper, salt, vinegar and olive oil; add squash. Toss until it's coated. Marinate it for 10 minutes.

Preheat outdoor grill to high heat. Oil the grate lightly.

On the preheated grill, put squash slices. Cook for 3 minutes per side till it turns light brown and until it's tender.

Grilled Green Garlic

Serv.: 4| **Prep.:** 5m | **Cook:** 30m

Ingredients:
- ✓ 1 bunch green garlic bulbs, tops sliced off
- ✓ 1 tablespoon olive oil, or as needed
- ✓ Sea salt and ground black pepper to taste (optional)

Directions: Set an outdoor grill to medium-high heat to preheat and lightly grease the grate.

On large sheets of aluminum foil, place up to 3 garlic bulbs per sheet. Spray olive oil lightly over bulbs, season with pepper and salt. Tightly wrap the foil around the bulbs.

On the top rack away from the flames, place the bulbs inside the preheated grill; cook for about 30 minutes or until the garlic cloves are butter-soft. Let cool until easy to handle. In a bowl, squeeze garlic from the bulb and use a fork to mash until spreadable.

Grilled Kale Salad

Serv.: 4| **Prep.:** 10m | **Cook:** 10m

Ingredients:
- ✓ Olive oil cooking spray
- ✓ 1 bunch kale, stems removed and discarded, leaves torn into bite-sized pieces
- ✓ 1/2 red onion, diced
- ✓ 2 carrots, cut into matchstick-sized pieces
- ✓ 2 jalapeno peppers, seeded and diced, or to taste

- ✓ 3 cloves garlic, chopped
- ✓ 1 tablespoon olive oil, or as needed
- ✓ Salt and ground black pepper to taste

Directions: Preheat a grill to medium heat. Oil grate lightly. Form aluminum foil sheet to shape of baking sheet. Spray cooking spray on.
In a bowl, mix pepper, salt, olive oil, garlic, jalapeno peppers, carrots, red onion and kale. Spread kale mixture on prepped aluminum foil.
On preheated grill, put aluminum foil baking sheet. Cook for 6-8 minutes till kale gets desired texture and reduces in size, tossing kale using tons.

GRILLED LEMON PEPPER CATFISH

Serv.: 2| **Prep.:** 20m | **Cook:** 15m

Ingredients:
- ✓ 5 lemons, juiced
- ✓ 1 tablespoon sea salt
- ✓ 3 large cloves garlic, minced
- ✓ 2 (8 ounce) fillets catfish
- ✓ 2 tablespoons lemon pepper seasoning (such as McCormick®)
- ✓ 2 tablespoons garlic and herb seasoning blend (such as Mrs. Dash®)
- ✓ 1 1/2 teaspoons Creole seasoning (such as Tony Chachere's®) (optional)
- ✓ 1 lemon, thinly sliced
- ✓ 1/4 cup shredded carrot
- ✓ 2 tablespoons chopped fresh parsley
- ✓ 1 lemon, quartered

Directions: Place juice from 5 lemons in a glass mixing bowl; stir in garlic and sea salt. Put in catfish fillets; cover and marinate for 1 to 4 hours in the fridge.
Turn the oven broilers to 400°F (205°C) to preheat; position the oven rack to the lowest level.
Take catfish out of the marinade, dripping off excess; pour off the rest of the marinade. Arrange fish fillets on a broiling pan; season with Creole seasoning, herb seasoning, garlic, and lemon pepper seasoning. Top fish with lemon slices. Broil fish for 12 to 15 minutes in the preheated oven until fork tender. If you want the edges of the fish darkened, turn the broiler on highest heat for

the last couple of minutes. Scatter top of fish fillets with parsley and shredded carrot to garnish. Serve fish with lemon wedges.

GRILLED OKRA SALAD

Serv.: 2| **Prep.:** 10m | **Cook:** 5m

Ingredients:
- ✓ 1/4 cup white wine vinegar
- ✓ 1 orange tomato, cubed
- ✓ 1/2 red onion, diced
- ✓ Salt to taste
- ✓ 16 pods fresh okra

Directions: Preheat outdoor grill to medium high heat; oil grate lightly. Mix salt, onion, tomato and vinegar in a bowl; put aside.
On preheated grill, cook okra for about 5 minutes till several black areas develop on skin. Toss okra with tomato mixture; serve.

GRILLED PHEASANT POPPERS

Serv.: 6| **Prep.:** 20m | **Cook:** 15m

Ingredients:
- ✓ 1 1/2 pounds pheasant breast
- ✓ 1 (4 ounce) jar sliced jalapeno peppers
- ✓ 12 slices bacon, cut into thirds
- ✓ 6 bamboo skewers, soaked in water for 20 minutes
- ✓ 36 toothpicks

Directions: Cut pheasant breast to 36 pieces. Put into bowl. Pour jalapeno peppers liquid on pheasant. Mix. Put aside. Marinate them for 20 minutes.
Preheat outdoor grill to medium heat. Oil the grate lightly.
Drain marinade from pheasant and discard. On every pheasant breast piece, put a jalapeno pepper slice. Use a 1/3 of strip of bacon to wrap. On each skewer, skewer 6 pheasant pieces.
On preheated grill, cook for 15-20 minutes, frequently turning, until bacon is crispy. Remove skewers from pheasant pieces. Put toothpicks on each piece. Serve.

HONEY FRUIT DESSERT

Serv.: 8| **Prep.:** 10m | **Cook:** 20m

Ingredients:
- ✓ 4 fresh plums, pitted and halved
- ✓ 2 fresh nectarines, pitted and halved
- ✓ 2 tablespoons honey

Directions: Set the oven for preheating to 425°F (220°C). Prepare a 9x13 inches baking pan and use an aluminum foil to line the pan, grease with cooking spray.
Arrange nectarines and plums, cut side up, on prepared baking pan.
Place in the preheated oven and let it bake for 18 to 20 minutes until softened. Pour the honey over fruit; put it back in the oven and continue to bake until golden brown for 2-3 minutes.

HONEY GINGER SHRIMP

Serv.: 4| **Prep.:** 10m | **Cook:** 10m

Ingredients:
- ✓ 2 tablespoons olive oil
- ✓ 1 tablespoon red pepper flakes
- ✓ 1 teaspoon chopped garlic
- ✓ 1/4 yellow onion, chopped
- ✓ 1 teaspoon ground ginger
- ✓ 1 teaspoon honey
- ✓ 1 pound medium shrimp - peeled and deveined
- ✓ Salt and pepper to taste

Directions: In a large skillet, heat red pepper flakes and olive oil over medium heat. Put in honey, ginger, garlic and onions. Cook while stirring until fragrant. Put in shrimp, cook until the shrimp are opaque and pink, stirring as needed, about 5 minutes. Serve right away.

HONEY LEMON GLAZED SALMON WITH SPINACH SAUTE

Serv.: 4| **Prep.:** 15m | **Cook:** 10m

Ingredients:
- ✓ 1 lemon
- ✓ 1/4 cup honey
- ✓ 1 pound salmon fillets
- ✓ Freshly ground Spice Islands® Black Pepper Adjustable Grinder
- ✓ 1 1/2 teaspoons Mazola® Corn Oil
- ✓ 1/2 cup thinly sliced red onions
- ✓ 2 cloves garlic, thinly sliced
- ✓ 1 (5 ounce) package fresh baby spinach
- ✓ 1/4 cup dry white wine
- ✓ 1/4 teaspoon Spice Islands® Crushed Red Pepper
- ✓ 1/8 teaspoon salt
- ✓ 1 tablespoon chopped, toasted pine nuts

Directions: Turn oven to 450°F to preheat. Grate zest from a lemon; put to one side. Take 1 tablespoon juice squeezed from the lemon and put into a small mixing bowl. Stir in honey and combine well. Line foil over a baking sheet; apply cooking spray over the foil. Arrange salmon fillets on a baking sheet. Liberally season fish with black pepper. Drizzle half of the honey mixture over salmon. Roast fish in the preheated oven until fish turns light brown and flakes easily for 10 to 12 minutes. Brush salmon with the remaining glaze if necessary. Broil fish on high heat on the last few minutes of cooking time for a browner glaze.
Heat oil over medium-high heat in a large nonstick skillet. Sauté garlic and onions in heated oil for 3 to 5 minutes. Stir in white wine and spinach. Sauté until most of the liquid has vaporized and spinach is wilted. Stir in salt, crushed red pepper, and 1 teaspoon lemon zest. Arrange spinach evenly atop salmon fillets and scatter pine nuts over. Serve right away.

HONEY LIME FRUIT SALAD

Serv.: 8| **Prep.:** 20m | **Cook:** 0

Ingredients:
- ✓ 2 large bananas, sliced
- ✓ 1 (16 ounce) package fresh strawberries, hulled and sliced
- ✓ 1/2 pound fresh blueberries
- ✓ 2 tablespoons honey

- ✓ 1 lime, juiced
- ✓ 1/3 cup pine nuts

Directions: In a bowl, mix in blueberries, strawberries and bananas. Toss them together with lime juice and honey, mix to coat the fruits. Top with pine nuts.

HONEY ROASTED CARROTS WITH CUMIN

Serv.: 4| **Prep.:** 10m | **Cook:** 30m

Ingredients:
- ✓ 1 (8 ounce) package baby carrots
- ✓ 1/4 cup honey
- ✓ 2 tablespoons olive oil
- ✓ 1/2 teaspoon ground cumin
- ✓ Salt and ground black pepper to taste

Directions: Set the oven to 220°C or 425°F.
In a big sealable plastic bag, add carrots, then put in black pepper, salt, cumin, olive oil and honey. Seal the bag and manipulate the contents until the carrots are coated thoroughly, then turn out into a baking dish.
In the preheated oven, roast for 30-40 minutes, until just softened or to your wanted degree of doneness.

HONEY TOMATOES

Serv.: 4| **Prep.:** 3m | **Cook:** 30m

Ingredients:
- ✓ 2 large tomatoes, each cut into 8 wedges
- ✓ 2 1/2 cups honey

Directions: Put tomatoes into a storage container or jar; pour honey over tomatoes. Chill for half an hour in the fridge. Take tomatoes out of the honey, and enjoy.

HONEY AND GINGER CHICKEN

Serv.: 6| **Prep.:** 20m | **Cook:** 15m

Ingredients:
- ✓ 2 tablespoons olive oil
- ✓ 2 large boneless, skinless chicken breasts, cubed
- ✓ 1/4 cup honey
- ✓ 2 tablespoons finely chopped ginger
- ✓ 2 red bell peppers, chopped
- ✓ 1 large onion, cut into 8 wedges
- ✓ 1 large head broccoli, cut into florets
- ✓ 1 cup peeled and cubed fresh pineapple
- ✓ 1/2 cup honey

Directions: Heat a frying pan or wok with olive oil over medium heat. Put in the ginger, chicken cubes and 1/4 cup of honey. Stir-fry the mixture for about 10 minutes or until the chicken turns golden brown. Mix in the remaining 1/2 cup of honey, broccoli, pineapple, bell peppers and onion. Cover the wok and cook the vegetables over medium-high heat for 5-10 minutes while stirring it once in a while until the vegetables are soft.

HONEY BALSAMIC CHICKEN

Serv.: 6| **Prep.:** 10m | **Cook:** 35m

Ingredients:
- ✓ 1/4 cup balsamic vinegar
- ✓ 1/4 cup olive oil
- ✓ 1/4 cup honey
- ✓ 1/2 teaspoon dried thyme
- ✓ 1/2 teaspoon dried rosemary
- ✓ 2 pounds bone-in chicken thighs, or more to taste
- ✓ Salt and pepper to taste

Directions: In a bowl, beat rosemary, thyme, honey, olive oil and balsamic vinegar till smooth; transfer the marinade into a resealable plastic bag. Season black pepper and salt on chicken thighs; add into the marinade in the plastic bag. Squeeze the bag to remove any air; seal. Marinate the chicken for 2-8 hours in the refrigerator.
Set the oven at 375°F (190°C) and start preheating. Pour the marinade and the chicken into a baking dish.
Bake for 35-40 minutes in the preheated oven till the juices run clear and the chicken is not pink in the bone anymore. An instant-read thermometer

should read 165°F (74°C) when inserted near the bone.

HONEY GLAZED CHINESE CHICKEN

Serv.: 6| **Prep.:** 2h | **Cook:** 1h

Ingredients:
- ✓ 1/2 cup Kikkoman Teriyaki Marinade Sauce
- ✓ 1/4 cup Kikkoman Hoisin Sauce
- ✓ 1/4 cup honey
- ✓ 2 1/2 pounds chicken drumsticks
- ✓ 1 green onion, thinly sliced

Directions: Mix first 3 ingredients. In a big plastic food storage bag, put over chicken; press air out of bag. Securely close top. Turn bag over a few times to coat all pieces well. Refrigerate, occasionally turning bag over, for 2 hours to overnight.
Bake chicken for 1 hour in a 350°F oven, flipping pieces and basting using pan juices once. Sprinkle green onion on then serve.

HOSHI SHIITAKE DASHI

Serv.: 4| **Prep.:** 5m | **Cook:** 5m

Ingredients:
- ✓ 4 cups water
- ✓ 4 dried shiitake mushrooms

Directions: In a saucepan, combine the water and mushrooms; let sit 10 minutes. Next, bring to a boil; remove from heat, let sit for another 20 minutes. Through a mesh strainer, filter the mixture before using.

MEDITERRANEAN LEMON CHICKEN

Serv.: 6| **Prep.:** 15m | **Cook:** 50m

Ingredients:
- ✓ 1 lemon
- ✓ 2 teaspoons dried oregano
- ✓ 3 cloves garlic, minced
- ✓ 1 tablespoon olive oil
- ✓ 1/4 teaspoon salt
- ✓ 1/4 teaspoon ground black pepper
- ✓ 6 chicken legs

Directions: Set the oven to 425°F or 220°C for preheating.
In a 9x13-inches baking dish, grate the peel from the lemon half. Squeeze the juice out from the lemon, about 1/4 cup of juice, and add it into the peel together with the pepper, oil, oregano, salt, and garlic. Stir the mixture until well blended. Remove and discard the skin from the chicken pieces. Coat the lemon mixture all over the chicken pieces. Arrange the chicken into the baking dish, bone-side up. Cover the dish and bake the chicken for 20 minutes. Flip the chicken and baste.
Adjust the heat to 400°F or 205°C. Bake the chicken while uncovered for 30 more minutes, basting the chicken every 10 minutes. Serve the chicken together with its pan juices.

MEDITERRANEAN SALMON

Serv.: 4| **Prep.:** 10m | **Cook:** 15m

Ingredients:
- ✓ 1/2 cup olive oil
- ✓ 1/4 cup balsamic vinegar
- ✓ 4 cloves garlic, pressed
- ✓ 4 (3 ounce) fillets salmon
- ✓ 1 tablespoon chopped fresh cilantro
- ✓ 1 tablespoon chopped fresh basil
- ✓ 1 1/2 teaspoons garlic salt

Directions: In a small bowl, combine together the balsamic vinegar and olive oil. Spread salmon fillets onto a shallow baking dish. Brush garlic over the fillets, and then spread the oil and vinegar on top of them flipping once to coat. Season with garlic salt, basil, and cilantro. Save to marinate for ten minutes.
Preheat the oven's broiler.
Put salmon approximately 6 inches away from the heat and broil for about 15 minutes, flipping once, or until fish is browned on each side and flaked easily with a fork. Baste often with sauce from the pan.

MEDITERRANEAN TWIST SALMON

Serv.: 2| **Prep.:** 10m | **Cook:** 20m

Ingredients:
Salmon:
- ✓ 1 teaspoon olive oil
- ✓ 2 (4 ounce) fillets salmon
Sauce:
- ✓ 2 tablespoons olive oil
- ✓ 1 clove garlic, minced
- ✓ 1/2 cup chopped tomatoes, or more to taste
- ✓ 1 tablespoon balsamic vinegar
- ✓ 6 fresh basil leaves, chopped

Directions: In a saucepan, put in 1 teaspoon of olive oil and let it heat up over medium heat setting. Put in the salmon and let it cook in hot oil for 5-7 minutes on every side until the fish meat can be flaked apart easily using a fork and it has been cooked thoroughly.

In another saucepan, put in 2 tablespoons of olive oil and let it heat up over medium heat setting then put in the garlic and sauté it for about 1 minute until you can smell the garlic aroma. Put in the tomatoes and let it cook for about 5 minutes until it is thoroughly heated. Add in the balsamic vinegar then followed by the basil. Let the tomato mixture cook for about 3 minutes while stirring it until the flavors have combined.

Transfer the cooked salmon onto a plate and spoon over the prepared tomato sauce.

KALE SALAD

Serv.: 6| **Prep.:** 30m | **Cook:** 0

Ingredients:
- ✓ 2 bunches fresh kale, cut into bite-size pieces
- ✓ 2 apples - peeled, cored, and diced
- ✓ 2 avocados - peeled, pitted, and diced
- ✓ 1 cup halved cherry tomatoes, or more to taste
- ✓ 1/2 red onion, diced
- ✓ 1/2 bunch fresh cilantro, chopped
Dressing:
- ✓ 3 tablespoons olive oil, or to taste
- ✓ 2 tablespoons apple cider vinegar, or to taste
- ✓ 1 large clove garlic, minced
- ✓ 1 pinch dried oregano, or to taste
- ✓ Salt and ground black pepper to taste

Directions: Combine cilantro, red onion, tomatoes, avocados, apples and kale into a bowl. Mix black pepper, salt, oregano, garlic, cider vinegar, olive oil in a different bowl to create a thick and smooth dressing. Toss the dressing with the kale mixture to have it fully coated.

MELITZANES IMAM

Serv.: 2| **Prep.:** 30m | **Cook:** 45m

Ingredients:
- ✓ 1 eggplant
- ✓ 1 (14.5 ounce) can diced tomatoes, drained
- ✓ 1 tablespoon tomato paste
- ✓ 1 medium onion, chopped
- ✓ 1 tablespoon minced garlic, or to taste
- ✓ 1 teaspoon ground cinnamon, or to taste
- ✓ 3 tablespoons olive oil
- ✓ Salt and pepper to taste

Directions: Set the oven to 175°C or 350°F.
Halve the eggplant lengthways and hollow out the halves to leave approximately a 1 cm. shell. Set aside the flesh from the insides for later use. Put the shells on a baking tray and drizzle a little olive oil over.
In the preheated oven, bake for about half an hour until softened.
While those are baking, chop the remaining eggplant into small pieces. In a big skillet, heat approximately 2 tbsp. olive oil on medium heat, then add garlic and onion. Cook and stir for several minutes. Put in the chopped eggplant, then cook and stir until softened. Stir in tomato paste and tomatoes until well blended, then simmer on low heat until the halves in the oven are ready.
Take the baked eggplant shells out of the oven, then scoop in the eggplant and tomato mixture. Sprinkle on top of each one with a little cinnamon and take them back to the oven. Bake for 30 minutes more or so.

MELON HEAVEN

Serv.: 6| **Prep.:** 20m | **Cook:**

Ingredients:
- ✓ 1 large ripe cantaloupe
- ✓ 2 quarts cold water
- ✓ 1 large honeydew melon

Directions: Shred the cantaloupe then put in a 2-qt. pitcher. Add water to the pitcher and keep in the refrigerator for overnight.
Form little balls out of the honeydew melon using a balling spoon. Then transfer the honeydew melon balls to the cantaloupe mixture just prior to serving.

MEXICAN TURKEY

Serv.: 4| **Prep.:** 10m | **Cook:** 15m

Ingredients:
- ✓ 1 teaspoon vegetable oil
- ✓ 1 onion, chopped
- ✓ 1 pound shredded cooked turkey
- ✓ 1 teaspoon garlic powder
- ✓ 1 large fresh tomato, chopped
- ✓ 1/2 cup water
- ✓ 1 tablespoon chopped fresh cilantro
- ✓ Salt and pepper to taste

Directions: In a skillet, heat oil over moderate heat, and cook onion till soft. Stir in turkey, and put in garlic powder to season. Mix in tomato. Add water, scatter cilantro on top, and add pepper and salt to season. Place cover on skillet, and let simmer for 5 minutes, or till heated completely.

- BOOK 2 -
PALEO DIET FOR WOMEN

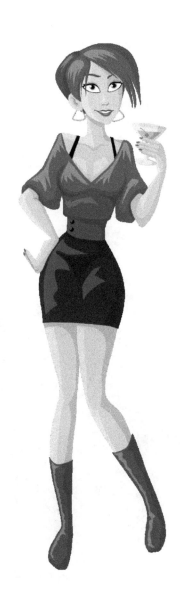

CRAWFISH IN RED SAUCE

Serv.: 10| Prep.: 25m | Cook: 50m

Ingredients:
- ✓ 3 tablespoons vegetable oil
- ✓ 1 tablespoon minced garlic
- ✓ 1 large onion, chopped
- ✓ 1/4 cup chopped green bell pepper
- ✓ 1/4 cup chopped celery
- ✓ 1 (8 ounce) can tomato sauce
- ✓ 1 (14.5 ounce) can whole peeled tomatoes, undrained and chopped
- ✓ 1/2 (14.5 ounce) can diced tomatoes with green chile peppers (such as RO*TEL®)
- ✓ Salt and pepper to taste
- ✓ 5 pounds cooked and peeled whole crawfish tails

Directions: Put vegetable oil in a large saucepan and heat it over medium heat. Mix in bell pepper, garlic, celery, and onion and cook for 10 minutes until the celery is tender and the onion is translucent. Stir in chopped tomatoes together with their juice, diced tomatoes, and tomato sauce. Season the mixture with salt and pepper to taste. Boil the mixture over medium-high heat. Decrease the heat and let it simmer for 30 minutes. Mix in crawfish tails. Simmer for 5-10 minutes until hot.

FRUIT SMOOTHIE

Serv.: 1| Prep.: 10m | Cook: 0

Ingredients:
- ✓ 1 1/2 cups crushed ice
- ✓ 1 banana, chopped
- ✓ 1 kiwi, peeled and chopped
- ✓ 1/2 cup chopped strawberries
- ✓ 1/2 cup chopped pineapple
- ✓ 1/4 cup cream of coconut
- ✓ 1 tablespoon coconut flakes for garnish

Directions: Using a blender, mix kiwi, pineapple, strawberries and banana together with ice and cream of coconut. Blend and mix until it becomes

smooth. Transfer it into the glass and decorate it with coconut flakes before serving.

CREOLE PORK SHANKS WITH SWEET POTATO GRAVY

Serv.: 4| Prep.: 25m | Cook: 6h

Ingredients:
- ✓ 2 sweet potatoes
- ✓ 1 teaspoon vegetable oil
- ✓ 4 pork shanks, cut in half
- ✓ 1/2 teaspoon ground black pepper
- ✓ 1/4 teaspoon cayenne pepper
- ✓ 1/4 cup olive oil
- ✓ 1 medium onion, chopped
- ✓ 3 celery ribs, chopped
- ✓ 1 small green bell pepper, chopped
- ✓ 4 garlic cloves, minced
- ✓ 4 cups Swanson® Chicken Broth, plus more if needed
- ✓ 2 (14.5 ounce) cans diced tomatoes
- ✓ 3 bay leaves
- ✓ 1 teaspoon dried thyme
- ✓ 1/4 teaspoon cayenne pepper
- ✓ 1/2 teaspoon black pepper

Directions: Preheat an oven to 175°C/350°F; rub vegetable oil on sweet potatoes. In aluminum foil, wrap.
In preheated oven, put sweet potatoes; bake for 1 hour till soft. Peel then cut into 1-in. chunks when cool enough to handle.
Season all sides of pork shanks with cayenne pepper and black pepper.
Heat olive oil in big skillet on medium-high heat; cook all sides of shanks for 10 minutes in total till all sides are nicely browned. Put pork shanks into slow cooker.
Sauté garlic, bell pepper, celery and onion in skillet, scraping browned bits from the bottom; cook on medium heat for 5 minutes till soft.
Mix diced tomatoes and 4 cups of Swanson® Chicken Broth in; boil. Add thyme and bay leaves; simmer for 10 minutes till mixture slightly reduces. Put mixture into slow cooker with pork shanks;

cook for 6 hours on high till tender. Put pork shanks onto a platter; to keep warm, tent with foil.

Take 1/2 veggies out of the cooking liquid; discard/keep for another use. Put all liquid and leftover veggies into a food processor/blender; put cooked sweet potato chunks in; process for 1 minute till smooth.

Add 2 tbsp. chicken broth at a time till you get your desired gravy consistency in case the gravy is too thick.

Put sweet potato gravy on top of pork shank servings.

CREOLO COCKTAIL

Serv.: 1| **Prep.:** 5m | **Cook:** 0

Ingredients:
- ✓ 1 lemon, cut into 4 wedges
- ✓ 5 leaves fresh mint
- ✓ 1/4 fluid ounce agave nectar
- ✓ 1 cup crushed ice
- ✓ 1 1/2 fluid ounces spiced rum
- ✓ 1 fluid ounce club soda, or as needed
- ✓ 1 sprig fresh mint

Directions: In a lowball glass, muddle together agave nectar, mint leaves and 3 lemon wedges until aromatic. Put in rum and crushed ice, then put club soda on top. Pour the mixture back froth into a cocktail shaker or mixing glass until mixed.

Serve in a lowball glass decorated with a lemon wedge and a sprig of fresh mint.

PORK SAUSAGE PATTIES WITH APRICOTS AND PISTACHIOS

Serv.: 4| **Prep.:** 20m | **Cook:** 12m

Ingredients:
- ✓ 1 1/2 pounds coarsely ground pork
- ✓ 2 teaspoons kosher salt
- ✓ 1 teaspoon black pepper
- ✓ 1 pinch cayenne pepper
- ✓ 1 pinch dried sage
- ✓ 1 teaspoon very finely sliced fresh sage leaves
- ✓ 1/4 cup chopped pistachio nuts

- ✓ 2 tablespoons diced dried apricots
- ✓ 1/2 pound caul fat

Directions: In the mixing bowl, whisk together apricots, pistachios, fresh sage, dried sage, cayenne pepper, pepper, salt, and sausage using a fork till just combined. Split into 4 parts and form into patties that are roughly three quarters in. in thickness.

Chop the caul fat into pieces that are roughly 2-3 in. bigger than the crepinette patty. Wrap the patty in caul fat with the ends tucked on the bottom. The patties should be covered entirely. If the caul fat pieces are small, overlap them to cover each patty entirely. Trim off any redundant caul fat, as you want. Add the patties onto the dish and use the plastic wrap to cover up; keep in the refrigerator overnight.

Heat 1 tbsp. of oil on medium heat in the skillet. Add the crepinettes smooth side facing downward into the pan. Allow to brown for 3 - 4 minutes per side. Blot some of rendered fat using the wadded up paper towel. Add in a splash of the white wine; cover up. Cook while covered till the inside of patties reaches 63 degrees C/145 degrees F in temperature, or 5 more minutes. Remove the cover and turn the crepinettes to coat along with pan brownings and to decrease some of the wine.

CRISPY PORK CARNITAS

Serv.: 6| **Prep.:** 15m | **Cook:** 3h40m

Ingredients:
- ✓ 3 pounds boneless pork butt (shoulder)
- ✓ 8 cloves garlic, peeled
- ✓ 1/4 cup olive oil
- ✓ 1 orange, juiced, orange parts of peel removed and sliced into thin strips
- ✓ 1 tablespoon kosher salt
- ✓ 2 bay leaves, torn in half
- ✓ 1 teaspoon ground black pepper
- ✓ 1 teaspoon ground cumin
- ✓ 3/4 teaspoon ground cinnamon
- ✓ 1/2 teaspoon Chinese 5-spice powder

Directions: Set oven to 135°C (or 275°F) and start preheating.

Skim fat off the pork; cube pork meat into 2" pieces and coarsely chop fat.

In a bowl, combine 5-spice powder, cinnamon, cumin, black pepper, bay leaves, salt, orange juice, orange peel, olive oil, garlic with pork until pork is thoroughly coated. Bring mixture to a 9x13" baking dish. Set the dish on a baking sheet and tightly wrap heavy-duty aluminum foil around.

Bake pork for 3 1/2 hours in prepared oven until pork is easily flaked with a fork.

Place oven rack in a 6"-distance away from the heat; start preheating the oven's broiler.

Set meat onto a colander placed over a bowl. Take out orange peels, bay leaves and garlic from baking dish and stream accumulated juices from the baking dish onto the meat placed in colander into the bowl. Take meat back to the baking dish and pour accumulated juices onto each piece of meat. Cook meat for 3 minutes in the prepared broiler. Pour more accumulated juices onto the meat and keep broiling for another 3-5 minutes until crisped. Bring pork to serving dish and top with more accumulated juices.

Crispy and Tender Baked Chicken Thighs

Serv.: 8 | **Prep.:** 10m | **Cook:** 1h

Ingredients:
Cooking spray:
✓ 8 bone-in chicken thighs with skin
✓ 1/4 teaspoon garlic salt
✓ 1/4 teaspoon onion salt
✓ 1/4 teaspoon dried oregano
✓ 1/4 teaspoon ground thyme
✓ 1/4 teaspoon paprika
✓ 1/4 teaspoon ground black pepper

Directions: Set oven to 350°F (175°C) to preheat. Line aluminum foil over a baking sheet and apply cooking spray all over.

Place chicken thighs on the prepared baking sheet.

In a small container with a lid, mix together pepper, paprika, thyme, oregano, onion salt, and garlic salt. Cover the container with a lid and shake until spices are well blended. Scatter spice mixture generously over chicken thighs.

Bake chicken for about 60 minutes in the preheated oven until no pink remain at the bones, chicken juices run clear, and skin is crispy. An instant-read thermometer pinned near the bone should register 165°F (74°C).

Crispy, Spicy Cauliflower Pancakes

Serv.: 12 | **Prep.:** 15m | **Cook:** 36m

Ingredients:
✓ 1 tablespoon coconut oil
✓ 1 teaspoon olive oil
✓ 2 cups grated cauliflower
✓ 2 tablespoons finely chopped onion
✓ 1 clove garlic, minced
✓ 1 cup 1% cottage cheese, drained
✓ 1/4 cup egg whites
✓ 1 tablespoon hot pepper sauce (such as Frank's RedHot®), or to taste
✓ 2 teaspoons dried parsley
✓ 1 teaspoon dried oregano
✓ 1/4 teaspoon garlic powder

Directions: Prepare the oven by preheating to 350°F (175°C). Use coconut oil to grease a 12-cup muffin tin.

Put the olive oil in a skillet over medium heat. Put in the garlic, onion, and cauliflower. Stir and cook for 6-8 minutes until the cauliflower turns slightly translucent and garlic and onions are tender. Transfer to a bowl allows it to cool.

In a blender, combine garlic powder, oregano, parsley, hot sauce, egg whites, and cottage cheese; blend until smooth. Place into the bowl of cauliflower mixture; blend fully. Scoop mixture equally into the greased muffin cups and push down so pancakes are flat and equal.

Place in the preheated oven and bake for approximately 30 minutes until tops and edges are crispy and golden.

CUBAN GOULASH

Serv.: 6| **Prep.:** 20m | **Cook:** 40m

Ingredients:
- ✓ 1 tablespoon vegetable oil
- ✓ 1 pound boneless pork roast, cubed
- ✓ 1 pound onions, diced
- ✓ 1 pound bananas, peeled and diced
- ✓ 1 (16 ounce) can diced tomatoes with juice
- ✓ Cayenne pepper to taste
- ✓ Salt and ground black pepper to taste

Directions: Over medium heat, heat oil in a large skillet, add pork and then brown on all sides. Stir in onions and then cook while stirring until tender. Combine the tomatoes with juice and bananas into the skillet. Heat to boil, decrease the heat to medium low and let simmer for 30 minutes while stirring often until the pork becomes very tender. Season with pepper, salt and cayenne pepper.

CURRIED BEEF

Serv.: 4| **Prep.:** 10m | **Cook:** 35m

Ingredients:
- ✓ 2 tablespoons vegetable oil
- ✓ 1 pound stew beef, cubed
- ✓ 1 1/2 teaspoons curry powder
- ✓ 1/2 teaspoon salt
- ✓ 1/2 teaspoon ground black pepper
- ✓ 2 tablespoons tomato paste
- ✓ 1/4 cup water
- ✓ 1 onion, chopped
- ✓ 2 stalks celery, chopped
- ✓ 1/2 cup raisins
- ✓ 1 apple - peeled, cored, and chopped

Directions: Heat the oil in a large skillet over medium heat. Place the meat in the hot oil and sauté until well browned on all sides. Sprinkle the curry powder, salt, and ground black pepper over the meat and stir well.
Beat water and tomato paste together in a small bowl, then mix the mixture into the skillet. Stir in raisins, celery, and onion, turn down the heat to low and simmer until the beef becomes tender, half an hour.
Mix the apple into the skillet and simmer until the sauce becomes thick and the apple becomes tender, 5 minutes longer.

CURRY SALMON WITH MANGO

Serv.: 4| **Prep.:** 15m | **Cook:** 15m

Ingredients:
- ✓ 1 (1 pound) fillet salmon fillet
- ✓ 1/4 cup avocado oil
- ✓ 1 teaspoon curry powder
- ✓ Salt to taste
- ✓ 1 mango - peeled, seeded, and diced
- ✓ 1/4 cup diced red onion
- ✓ 1 small serrano pepper, diced
- ✓ 1 small bunch cilantro leaves
- ✓ 1 lime

Directions: Set oven to 400°F or 200°C. Use aluminum foil to line cookie sheet.
Put the salmon in cookie sheet and cover salmon with the foil. Crumple the edges to seal.
Bake for about 15 minutes until fish flakes easily using fork.
Meanwhile, combine curry powder, avocado oil and salt in a small bowl. Pour dressing over the salmon and top with red onion, serrano pepper and diced mango. Before serving, squeeze lime and sprinkle cilantro on top.

CZECH CABBAGE DISH

Serv.: 10| **Prep.:** 20m | **Cook:** 10m

Ingredients:
- ✓ 1 large head cabbage, shredded
- ✓ 1/4 pound bacon, chopped
- ✓ 1 tablespoon vegetable oil
- ✓ 1 small onion, chopped
- ✓ 1 stalk celery, chopped
- ✓ 1/4 cup chopped green bell pepper
- ✓ 3 tablespoons white vinegar
- ✓ 1/2 teaspoon salt

✓ 1 teaspoon black pepper

Directions: Boil a large pot filled with lightly salted water and then blanche the cabbage into the water briefly. Remove them from water and drain them right away.

Cook the bacon in a large skillet over medium heat until brown and opaque. Remove from the heat and let it drain on paper towels.

Discard all the bacon grease except for 1 tbsp. of it. Add 1 tbsp. of vegetable oil to the skillet. Heat the oil over medium heat. Add the bell pepper, celery, and onion. Cook until crisp-tender.

Mix the bacon, salt, pepper, prepared cabbage, vinegar, and sautéed vegetable mix with oil in a large bowl. Toss the mixture well and serve while warm. You can also chill the mixture and serve it later.

SHREDDED BEEF

Serv.: 4| **Prep.:** 10m | **Cook:** 5h

Ingredients:
✓ 1 1/2 pounds rump roast
✓ 1 1/4 cups water
✓ Garlic powder, or to taste
✓ Salt and ground black pepper to taste

Directions: Generously season rump roast with pepper, salt and garlic powder; place into the crock of a slow cooker. Pour the water into the crock. Cook for 5 hours on high. Take the roast away onto a cutting board; use 2 forks to shred.

BEST HAROSET

Serv.: 4| **Prep.:** 10m | **Cook:** 0

Ingredients:
✓ 3 apples - peeled, cored, and diced
✓ 1 cup walnuts, chopped
✓ 1 cup pecans, chopped
✓ 1 cup kosher red wine
✓ 1 teaspoon cinnamon

Directions: In a big bowl, mix wine, pecans, walnuts and apples together. Use cinnamon to season. Stir the mixture and put it in the refrigerator for about 30 minutes until chilled.

ROAST PORK PUERTO RICAN STYLE

Serv.: 8| **Prep.:** 15m | **Cook:** 4h

Ingredients:
✓ 1/4 cup olive oil
✓ 3 tablespoons white vinegar
✓ 10 cloves garlic, or more to taste
✓ 2 tablespoons dried oregano
✓ 1 tablespoon salt
✓ 1 1/2 teaspoons ground black pepper
✓ 5 pounds pork shoulder, trimmed of excess fat

Directions: In a mortar and pestle, mix black pepper, salt, oregano, garlic, vinegar and olive oil together before mashing them up to a paste. Use a little knife to cut some slits deep into the pork then insert the paste into slits. Place any leftover paste atop pork, rubbing it in. Put the pork into a plastic roasting bag then set it on a rack inside of a roasting pan. Leave it marinating for a minimum of 8 hours up to 48 hours.

After getting the pork out from the fridge, remove the cover and let it cool down for an hour or two hours until it's at room temperature.

Preheat the oven to 300°F (150°C).

Put the meat into the preheated oven, roasting for around 2 hours with the skin side facing down until it becomes a nice golden brown. Turn the pork around. Proceed to roast with the skin side up for about 2-4 hours until the juices start running clear. It's done when the instant-read thermometer reads a minimum of 145°F (63°C) when put into the middle of the pork. If desired, serve with sweet plantains, salad or beans and rice.

DARK CHOCOLATE ALMOND ROCKS

Serv.: 20| **Prep.:** 10m | **Cook:** 8m

Ingredients:
✓ 1/2 cup almonds, crushed into chunks

✓ 7 ounces dark chocolate chips (50% cacao)

Directions: In big skillet, spread almonds; toast for 3-5 minutes till starting to brown on medium heat. Put almonds in bowl.

In top of double boiler above simmering water, melt chocolate, frequently mixing and scraping side down to avoid scorching for 5 minutes; take off heat. Put almonds in; mix till coated evenly.

On waxed paper-lined plate, drop spoonfuls of chocolate-almond mixture.

Chill for 10 minutes till set.

DARK CHOCOLATE ESPRESSO PALEO MUG CAKE

Serv.: 1| **Prep.:** 5m | **Cook:** 2m

Ingredients:
✓ 4 ounces dark chocolate chips
✓ 1 tablespoon coconut oil
✓ 2 tablespoons water
✓ 1 tablespoon blanched almond flour
✓ 1 tablespoon coconut flour
✓ 1 pinch baking soda
✓ 1 egg
✓ 1 tablespoon brewed espresso

Directions: In a microwave-safe mug, mix the coconut oil and chocolate chips. Let it heat in the microwave for about 30 seconds, until it melts. Whisk the baking soda, coconut flour, almond flour and water into the chocolate mixture, until well blended. Add brewed espresso and egg, then whisk until it becomes smooth.

Let it heat it in the microwave for about 90 seconds, until the cake is cooked through. Allow it to cool for about 2 minutes prior to serving.

DASHI STOCK

Serv.: 8| **Prep.:** 5m | **Cook:** 5m

Ingredients:
✓ 1 ounce dashi Kombu
✓ 1 quart water

✓ 1/2 cup bonito flakes

Directions: Use a paper towel to clean any dirt from the kombu, but be careful not to scuff the white powdery deposits on seaweed. In a saucepan, put water and the kombu, allow to soak for about 30 minutes to get softened.

Next, remove the seaweed from the water, trim some lengthways splits into the leaf. Put them back into the water and boil. When the water begins to boil, take the seaweed out to prevent the stock from getting bitter.

Stir the bonito flakes into the kombu-flavored broth, boil again, then remove the pan from the heat. Let the water cool down. Once the bonito flakes have sunk to the bottom, use a coffee filter or a strainer lined with cheesecloth to strain the dashi.

ROAST PORK FOR TACOS

Serv.: 12| **Prep.:** 15m | **Cook:** 4h

Ingredients:
✓ 4 pounds pork shoulder roast
✓ 2 (4 ounce) cans diced green chilies, drained
✓ 1/4 cup chili powder
✓ 1 teaspoon dried oregano
✓ 1 teaspoon taco seasoning
✓ 2 teaspoons minced garlic
✓ 1 1/2 teaspoons salt, or to taste

Directions: Set the oven to 300 degrees F (150 degrees C) to preheat.

Place roast atop a big piece of aluminum foil. Stir together garlic, taco seasoning, oregano, chili powder, and green chiles together in a small bowl; rub the mixture on the roast. Wrap the roast in the foil to completely cover it, using more foil if needed. Put it on a roasting rack set in a baking dish. Otherwise, you can just place a cookie sheet on an oven rack below to catch leaks.

Roast in prepared oven until the meat falls apart, around 3 1/2-4 hours. Cook the roast until it reaches a minimum of 145 degrees F or 63 degrees C. Take out of the oven and use 2 forks to shred the roast into small pieces, season to taste with salt.

Deep Fried Salt and Pepper Shrimp

Serv.: 8 | Prep.: 15m | Cook: 15m

Ingredients:
- ✓ 1 pound large shrimp in shells, peeled and deveined
- ✓ 3/4 teaspoon sea salt (such as Diamond Crystal®)
- ✓ 1/2 teaspoon freshly ground black pepper
- ✓ 1/2 teaspoon Chinese 5-spice powder
- ✓ 4 cups vegetable oil for frying

Directions: Cut off the hard pointed area right above the tail and the feathery legs of each shrimp. Rinse the shrimp; dry thoroughly.
In a small bowl, mix together 5-spice powder, pepper and salt.
In a heavy pot or a wok over high heat, heat oil till your deep fry thermometer attains 400°F (200°C). Cook the shrimp in the hot oil, around 5 per batch, for around 1 minute, or till the shrimp are cooked through and bright pink. Using a slotted spoon, take the shrimp away; remove onto a plate lined with paper towels. Turn the oil temperature back to 400°F (200°C) before each new batch.
Pour off the oil in the wok; place the wok over medium-high heat; put in the spice mix and the deep-fried shrimp; cook while stirring constantly for 30 seconds to 1 minute, or till fragrant.

Deep Fried Turkey

Serv.: 16 | Prep.: 30m | Cook: 45m

Ingredients:
- ✓ 3 gallons peanut oil for frying, or as needed
- ✓ 1 (12 pound) whole turkey, neck and giblets removed
- ✓ 1/4 cup Creole seasoning
- ✓ 1 white onion

Directions: Preheat oil to 400 degrees F (200 degrees C) in a big turkey fryer or a stockpot. Make sure not to fill the pot with too much oil or it will spill. Prepare a big platter and line it with paper towels or food-safe paper bags. Pat the rinsed turkey with paper towels until thoroughly dry. Massage the outside and cavity of the bird with Creole seasoning. See to it that the neck hole has a two-inch opening to ensure that the oil will reach the inside of the turkey. Put the turkey and whole onions in the drain basket, positioning the turkey neck end first. Carefully submerge the basket into the hot oil, completely submerging the turkey. Fry the turkey for 45 minutes or 3 1/2 minutes per pound, make sure that the oil stays at 350 degrees F (175 degrees C) throughout the cooking process. Slowly and carefully lift the basket from oil and drain the turkey. Thermometer inserted inside thickest area of thigh should read 180 degrees F (80 degrees C). Drain excess oil on prepared platter.

Deep Fried Turkey Breast

Serv.: 12 | Prep.: 5m | Cook: 25m

Ingredients:
- ✓ 2 tablespoons sea salt
- ✓ 1 tablespoon red pepper flakes
- ✓ 1 tablespoon freshly ground black pepper
- ✓ 1 tablespoon granulated garlic
- ✓ 1 tablespoon chili powder
- ✓ 1 (7 pound) turkey breast
- ✓ 2 gallons canola oil for frying

Directions: In a plastic container with a matching lid, combine the red pepper flakes, chili powder, granulated garlic, sea salt, and black pepper. Seal the container with its lid and shake until the seasonings are well-combined.
Rub the spice mixture all over the turkey breast until well-coated. Use an aluminum foil to wrap the breast; refrigerate for 24 hours.
Get the breast from the refrigerator and allow it to stand at room temperature.
Meanwhile, heat the oil in a pot with a lid (enough to hold the oil and breast to 325°F or 165°C).
Add the breast into the hot oil. Cover the pot with its lid. Fry the turkey for 25 minutes until its juices run clear and the turkey is no longer pinkish in the center. Make sure that the inserted instant-read thermometer into the turkey's center should read at least 165°F (74°C).

DELICIOUS SWEET POTATO FRIES

Serv.: 2| **Prep.:** 10m | **Cook:** 20m

Ingredients:
- ✓ 2 sweet potatoes, peeled and cut into 1/2-inch slices
- ✓ 1 tablespoon coconut oil, melted
- ✓ 1 teaspoon ground cumin
- ✓ 1/2 teaspoon garlic powder
- ✓ Salt and ground black pepper to taste
- ✓ 1/2 teaspoon paprika
- ✓ 2 tablespoons chopped fresh cilantro (optional)

Directions: Preheat the oven to 230°C or 450°F.
Onto a baking sheet, lay sweet potatoes. Sprinkle coconut oil on top of sweet potatoes; season with pepper, salt, garlic powder and cumin.
In the prepped oven, bake for 20 to 25 minutes till soft in the middle, flipping from time to time. Jazz up with cilantro and paprika.

DELICIOUS AND EASY PRIME RIB

Serv.: 14| **Prep.:** 15m | **Cook:** 3h30m

Ingredients:
- ✓ 1 (7 pound) bone-in prime rib, trimmed and retied to the bone
- ✓ 8 cloves garlic
- ✓ 2 tablespoons olive oil
- ✓ 2 teaspoons kosher salt
- ✓ 2 teaspoons freshly ground black pepper
- ✓ 1 ounce fresh rosemary, or to taste
- ✓ 1 ounce fresh thyme, or to taste

Directions: Start preheating the oven at 350°F (175°C).
Cut several slits into the top of prime rib; press garlic cloves into slits. Brush olive oil over the prime rib and flavor with pepper and salt. Place thyme sprigs and rosemary sprigs atop prime rib and put into a roasting pan.
Bake in the prepared oven for 3 1/2 to 4 hours until the outside is browned and the center is pink. An instant-read thermometer should show at least

125°F (52°C) when inserted into the center. Let the prime rib rest for 15 minutes before cutting.

FISH BAKED IN A SALT CRUST

Serv.: 4| **Prep.:** 30m | **Cook:** 30m

Ingredients:
- ✓ 2 pounds salt
- ✓ 7 bay leaves
- ✓ 2 pounds whole rainbow trout, gutted and cleaned, heads and tails still on
- ✓ 2 sprigs fresh cilantro, or more to taste
- ✓ 2 sprigs fresh parsley, or more to taste
- ✓ 2 sprigs fresh dill, or more to taste

Directions: Preheat the oven to 200 degrees C/400 degrees F. Line aluminum foil on a baking sheet.
Spread 1/4 - 1/2-lb. salt on aluminum foil to around the same shape as the fish. Put bay leaves on salt. Put fish on top. Stuff dill, parsley and cilantro into fish cavity. Firmly pack down leftover salt on fish. Leave tail and head exposed.
Bake in preheated oven for 30 minutes until salt crust becomes golden.
Remove fish from oven. Crack open salt crust carefully. Remove the top. Peel off fish skin to expose flesh. Use a spatula/fish knife to lift top fillet off the bones. In one piece, remove bones by lifting from the tail then pull upwards towards the head. Lift bottom fillet out with a spatula/knife.

TILAPIA FILIPINO SOUR BROTH DISH

Serv.: 4| **Prep.:** 5m | **Cook:** 10m

Ingredients:
- ✓ 1/2 pound tilapia fillets, cut into chunks
- ✓ 1 small head bok choy, chopped
- ✓ 2 medium tomatoes, cut into chunks
- ✓ 1 cup thinly sliced daikon radish
- ✓ 1/4 cup tamarind paste
- ✓ 3 cups water
- ✓ 2 dried red chile peppers (optional)

Directions: Mix radish, tomatoes, bok choy, and tilapia in a medium pot. Mix water and tamarind paste; add into the pot. Mix in the chili peppers if you want. Make it boil then cook for 5 minutes, or just until the fish is cooked well. Even fish that is frozen will be cooked in less than ten minutes. Keep from overcooking or else the fish will fall apart. Scoop into bowls to serve.

FLAT IRON STEAK

Serv.: 2| **Prep.:** 5m | **Cook:** 6m

Ingredients:
- ✓ 2 (8 ounce) flat iron steaks
- ✓ 1/2 teaspoon lemon pepper seasoning, or to taste
- ✓ 1/2 teaspoon onion powder, or to taste
- ✓ 1/2 teaspoon garlic powder, or to taste

Directions: Sprinkle garlic powder, onion powder and lemon pepper on both sides of the steak to season. Use plastic wrap to wrap and marinate in the refrigerator for at least 2 hours.
Set the grill to medium-high heat to preheat and let the steaks to come to room temperature. Remove wrap and put on the prepared grill. Cook to the degree of doneness you prefer, about 3 minutes on each side for medium rare. Before serving, let steaks sit for a few minutes.

FLAT IRON STEAK WITH MUSHROOMS

Serv.: 3| **Prep.:** 15m | **Cook:** 15m

Ingredients:
- ✓ 3 tablespoons vegetable oil
- ✓ Salt and pepper to taste
- ✓ 3 (6 ounce) flat iron steaks
- ✓ 3 shallots, thinly sliced
- ✓ 6 cloves garlic, peeled
- ✓ 4 cups sliced white mushrooms
- ✓ 1/4 cup balsamic vinegar
- ✓ 3/4 cup full-bodied red wine

Directions: Set the oven at 350°F (175°C) and start preheating.
In a large skillet over medium heat, heat oil. Slice flat iron steak into individual portions if necessary. Season both sides with pepper and salt. Fry the

steaks for 2-3 minutes on each side, till well-browned on both sides. Take away from the skillet; place on an oven-proof dish. Put the steaks into the oven; continue cooking.
Put whole cloves of garlic and shallots into the hot skillet. Cook while stirring over medium heat till the shallots begin to brown. Put in mushrooms; cook while stirring for 5-10 minutes, or till they shrink some.
Pour in balsamic vinegar; stir to discard any browned bits on the bottom of the skillet. Transfer in red wine; simmer over medium heat for a few minutes.
Transfer the steaks back to the skillet; cook for around 5 minutes if at all, or till the internal temperature registers 135-140°F (60°C). Take the whole pan away from the heat; allow to sit to reach your desired doneness, or till the steaks attain an internal temperature of 145°F (63°C).

FLOURLESS CREPE TORTILLAS

Serv.: 9| **Prep.:** 10m | **Cook:** 1m

Ingredients:
- ✓ 2 tablespoons water
- ✓ 2 teaspoons ghee (clarified butter), melted
- ✓ 4 eggs
- ✓ 1/2 cup tapioca flour
- ✓ 2 teaspoons coconut flour
- ✓ 1 pinch sea salt

Directions: Combine ghee and water together in a bowl. Whisk in egg until frothy. Add coconut flour, sea salt, and tapioca flour and mix until smooth. Place an 8-inches nonstick skillet over medium-low heat. Drop 2 tbsp. of the batter into the hot skillet and slowly swirl the skillet to coat the bottom evenly. Let it cook for 30 seconds. Flip it over and cook the other side for another 30 seconds. Place it into a plate. Do the same with the remaining batter.

FLOURLESS DOUBLE CHOCOLATE CHIP ZUCCHINI MUFFINS

Serv.: 8| **Prep.:** 30m | **Cook:** 25m

Ingredients:

- ✓ 1/2 cup almond butter
- ✓ 1 ripe banana, mashed
- ✓ 1/4 cup unsweetened cocoa powder
- ✓ 2 tablespoons ground flax seeds
- ✓ 1 tablespoon honey
- ✓ 1 teaspoon vanilla extract
- ✓ 1/2 teaspoon baking soda
- ✓ 1 cup finely grated zucchini, excess moisture squeezed out
- ✓ 1/4 cup semisweet chocolate chips
- ✓ 1/4 cup bittersweet chocolate chips, or to taste

Directions: Set the oven to 375°F or 190°C for preheating. Use an aluminum foil liners to line the muffin cups.

In a bowl, combine the banana, ground flax seeds, vanilla extract, baking soda, honey, cocoa powder, and almond butter until the batter is well-blended. Fold in semisweet chocolate chips and zucchini. Spoon the batter into the prepared muffin cups. Top each cups with bittersweet chocolate chips. Allow them to bake inside the preheated oven for 25 minutes until an inserted toothpick on its center comes out clean. Transfer muffins on a wire rack to cool completely.

FOOLPROOF RIB ROAST

Serv.: 6| **Prep.:** 5m | **Cook:** 5h

Ingredients:

- ✓ 1 (5 pound) standing beef rib roast
- ✓ 2 teaspoons salt
- ✓ 1 teaspoon ground black pepper
- ✓ 1 teaspoon garlic powder

Directions: Let the roast sit in room temperature for not less than 1 hour.

Preheat your oven to 375°F (190°C). In a small cup, mix the pepper, garlic powder and salt together. Put the roast onto the wire rack in the roasting pan, fat side facing up and rib side facing down. Massage the roast with the prepared seasoning. Put in preheated oven and let it roast for 1 hour. Switch off the oven and don't take out the roast.

Keep the oven door closed. Keep the roast inside the oven for 3 hours. Switch the oven back on at 375°F (190°C) temperature to reheat the roast 30-40 minutes before it's time to serve. The temperature inside the oven should not be less than 145°F (62°C). Take the roast out from the oven and let it sit for 10 minutes before slicing for serving.

FOOLPROOF ROSEMARY CHICKEN WINGS

Serv.: 2| **Prep.:** 20m | **Cook:** 40m

Ingredients:

- ✓ 1 1/2 pounds chicken wings, cut apart at joints, wing tips discarded
- ✓ 10 sprigs rosemary
- ✓ 1/2 whole head garlic, separated into cloves - cloves unpeeled and quartered
- ✓ 1 tablespoon olive oil, or as needed
- ✓ 1 teaspoon lemon pepper
- ✓ 1 teaspoon seasoned salt, or to taste

Directions: Turn the oven to 350°F (175°C) to preheat. On a broiler-proof baking sheet, place garlic cloves, rosemary, and chicken wings; ensure that they don't touch each other. Drizzle over the garlic and chicken with olive oil. Use seasoned salt and lemon pepper to season all sides of the wings. Bake for 35-40 minutes in the preheated oven until the juices run clear and around the bone of the chicken meat is not pink anymore, flipping the wings 1 time when they have cooked for 1/2 of the time. An instant-read thermometer should display a minimum of 160°F (70°C) when you insert it into the thickest sections of a wing.

Remove the baking sheet from the oven and turn the oven's broiler to High. Take the rosemary and garlic from the sheet and put aside. Flip the wings again.

Broil the wings for 5 minutes until turning golden brown. Use garlic and rosemary sprigs to garnish and enjoy.

July Salad

Serv.: 15 | **Prep.:** 10m | **Cook:** 0

Ingredients:
- ✓ 1 cup blueberries
- ✓ 1 cup sliced strawberries
- ✓ 1 cup chopped watermelon
- ✓ 1 cup red grapes
- ✓ 1 cup shredded coconut

Directions: In a bowl, combine grapes, watermelon, strawberries and blueberries then place in coconut.

Fragrant Lemon Chicken

Serv.: 6 | **Prep.:** 20m | **Cook:** 6-8h

Ingredients:
- ✓ 1 apple - peeled, cored and quartered
- ✓ 1 stalk celery with leaves, chopped
- ✓ 1 (3 pound) whole chicken
- ✓ Salt to taste
- ✓ Ground black pepper to taste
- ✓ 1 onion, chopped
- ✓ 1/2 teaspoon dried rosemary, crushed
- ✓ 1 lemon, zested and juiced
- ✓ 1 cup hot water

Directions: Rub pepper and salt on the skin of the chicken, then put celery and apple inside the chicken. Put the chicken in the slow cooker. Sprinkle chicken with lemon juice and zest, rosemary, and chopped onion. Add 1 cup of hot water into the slow cooker.
Cook, covered, on High for 1 hour. Change to low and cook for 6 to 8 hours, basting a few times.

Chopped Salsa

Serv.: 16 | **Prep.:** 25m | **Cook:** 0

Ingredients:
- ✓ 7 roma (plum) tomato, seeded and diced

- ✓ 6 cloves garlic, minced
- ✓ 6 jalapeno peppers, seeds and ribs removed, minced
- ✓ 1 small red onion, finely chopped
- ✓ 1 cup finely chopped cabbage
- ✓ 1 bunch fresh cilantro, chopped
- ✓ 1/3 cup fresh lime juice
- ✓ Salt to taste

Directions: In a big bowl, mix together lime juice, cilantro, cabbage, red onion, jalapenos, garlic and tomatoes. Season with salt to taste and chill for a couple of hours before serving.

Famous Spaghetti Sauce

Serv.: 8 | **Prep.:** 15m | **Cook:** 30m

Ingredients:
- ✓ 1 tablespoon olive oil
- ✓ 1 onion, chopped
- ✓ 1 green bell pepper, chopped
- ✓ 3 cloves garlic, minced
- ✓ 4 fresh mushrooms, sliced
- ✓ 1 pound ground turkey
- ✓ 1 pinch dried basil
- ✓ 1 pinch dried oregano
- ✓ Ground black pepper to taste
- ✓ 1 (14.5 ounce) can stewed tomatoes
- ✓ 2 (15 ounce) cans tomato sauce
- ✓ 1 (6 ounce) can tomato paste

Directions: The first part of this dish is simply sautéing garlic, green bell pepper, and onions together in olive oil in a big skillet over medium heat until the bell pepper is tender and onions are translucent. Put in the ground black pepper, oregano, basil, ground turkey, and mushrooms; fry while stirring frequently until the turkey is cooked. To the same pan you used for the first part, add the can of stewed tomatoes with the liquid. Lower the heat once you've added this and allow it to simmer until the tomatoes turn soft and start to fall apart. Put in tomato sauce and stir; thicken it by adding tomato paste. Turn the heat down to very low and allow the sauce to simmer for 15 minutes. Serve this with your preferred pasta.

FRENCH FRY SEASONING

Serv.: 5 | **Prep.:** 5m | **Cook:** 0

Ingredients:
- ✓ 2 teaspoons garlic salt
- ✓ 2 teaspoons onion salt
- ✓ 2 teaspoons salt
- ✓ 2 teaspoons ground paprika

Directions: In a bowl, mix together paprika, salt, onion salt and garlic salt. Turn into a zippered container to store.

FRENCH CANADIAN GORTON PORK SPREAD

Serv.: 16 | **Prep.:** 5m | **Cook:** 1h10m

Ingredients:
- ✓ 1 pound lean pork butt, cut into pieces
- ✓ 1 onion, chopped
- ✓ 1/2 teaspoon ground cinnamon
- ✓ 1/4 teaspoon ground cloves
- ✓ Salt and black pepper to taste

Directions: Get a saucepan then put the onion, cinnamon, pork and clove then add pepper and salt to taste. Add the water enough to cover meat. Turn on the stove to high heat, then minimize heat to medium-low and cover the saucepan for about 1 hour to cook until water has nearly absorbed. Occasionally stir to make the pork cook evenly. Make the pork into thin strands using a potato masher or wire whisk then remove the excess liquid and scoop out the gorton into a serving bowl. Place in the refrigerator until cold. Then serve.

GINGER CABBAGE PATCH SMOOTHIE

Serv.: 2 | **Prep.:** 10m | **Cook:**

Ingredients:
- ✓ 1 cup roughly chopped cabbage
- ✓ 1 cup red grapes
- ✓ 1 red apple, cored and chopped
- ✓ 1 large carrot, peeled and chopped
- ✓ 1/2 cup water
- ✓ 1/2 cup ice cubes
- ✓ 1 tablespoon chopped fresh ginger

Directions: Combine carrot, ginger, grapes, cabbage, ice cubes, water, and apple in a blender. Blend until the mixture is smooth.

GINGER SESAME SALMON

Serv.: 4 | **Prep.:** | **Cook:** 20m

Ingredients:
- ✓ 4 thin onion slices, separated into rings
- ✓ 2 sheets (12x18-inches each) Reynolds Wrap® Non-Stick Foil
- ✓ 2 medium carrots, cut into julienne strips or shredded
- ✓ 4 (4 ounce) salmon fillets, thawed
- ✓ 2 teaspoons grated fresh ginger
- ✓ 2 tablespoons seasoned rice vinegar
- ✓ 1 teaspoon sesame oil
- ✓ Salt and pepper to taste
- ✓ Fresh spinach leaves

Directions: Set grill to medium-high heat or preheat oven to 450°F.
Place 1/4 of onion slices and carrots in the center of each sheet Reynolds Wrap® nonstick foil. Lay salmon atop vegetables. Scatter ginger over salmon; drizzle with oil and vinegar. Scatter pepper and salt on top to season.
Bring the foil sides up. Double fold ends and top to seal packet, leaving space for heat circulation inside. Do the same with the remaining foil, making 4 packets in total.
Bake in the preheated oven on a cookie sheet, 16 to 20 minutes.
Or, grill in a covered grill for 14 to 16 minutes.
Serve carrots and salmon over a bed of spinach. If desired, sprinkle top with extra seasoned rice vinegar.

GINGER AND LIME SALMON

Serv.: 6 | **Prep.:** 15m | **Cook:** 15m

Ingredients:
- ✓ 1 (1 1/2-pound) salmon fillet
- ✓ 1 tablespoon olive oil
- ✓ 1 teaspoon seafood seasoning (such as Old Bay®)
- ✓ 1 teaspoon ground black pepper
- ✓ 1 (1 inch) piece fresh ginger root, peeled and thinly sliced
- ✓ 6 cloves garlic, minced
- ✓ 1 lime, thinly sliced

Directions: Position oven rack approximately 6 to 8 inches away from the heat source and preheat broiler; set oven's broiler to Low setting if there is. Line aluminum foil over a baking sheet.
Arrange salmon on the prepared baking sheet, skin side down; rub olive oil over the salmon. Season fish with black pepper and seafood seasoning.
Place ginger slices on top of salmon and scatter garlic over. Arrange lime slices over ginger-garlic layer.
Broil salmon for about 10 minutes until heated through and starting to turn opaque; watch carefully. Turn broiler to high setting if there is; keep broiling for 5 to 10 minutes longer or until salmon is thoroughly cooked and easily flaked using a fork.

GLUTEN FREE SHAKE AND BAKE ALMOND CHICKEN

Serv.: 4 | **Prep.:** 10m | **Cook:** 25m

Ingredients:
- ✓ 1/2 cup almond meal
- ✓ 1 teaspoon ground paprika
- ✓ 1 teaspoon sea salt
- ✓ 1 teaspoon ground black pepper
- ✓ 4 skinless, boneless chicken thighs

Directions: Preheat an oven to 175 °C or 350 °F.
In a resealable bag, mix black pepper, sea salt, paprika and almond meal together. Into the bag, place every thigh of chicken, one by one; seal the bag and shake till equally coated. In glass baking dish, put the chicken.
In the prepped oven, bake for 25 minutes to half an hour till juices run clear and not pink anymore in the middle. An inserted instant-read thermometer into the middle should register at minimum of 74 °C or 165 °F.

GOAN PORK VINDALOO

Serv.: 8 | **Prep.:** 30m | **Cook:** 1h25m

Ingredients:
- ✓ 16 dried Kashmiri chile peppers, stemmed and seeded
- ✓ 1 (1 inch) piece cinnamon stick
- ✓ 1 teaspoon cumin seeds
- ✓ 6 whole cloves
- ✓ 1/2 teaspoon whole black peppercorns
- ✓ 1/2 teaspoon ground turmeric
- ✓ 1 tablespoon white vinegar
- ✓ Salt to taste
- ✓ 2 pounds boneless pork loin roast, trimmed and cut into 1-inch cubes
- ✓ 1/4 cup vegetable oil
- ✓ 4 onions, chopped
- ✓ 10 cloves garlic, minced, or more to taste
- ✓ 1 (2 inch) piece fresh ginger root, minced
- ✓ 2 cups boiling water
- ✓ 2 green chile peppers, seeded and cut into strips
- ✓ 1/4 cup white vinegar

Directions: Using an electric coffee grinder or a mortar and pestle, grind turmeric, peppercorns, clove, cumin, cinnamon stick and Kashmiri chills till spices is smoothly ground. To make a smooth paste, combine with a tablespoon white vinegar. Season with salt to taste.
With the vinegar-spice paste, stir cubes of pork in a bowl till evenly coated. Put on plastic wrap to cover the bowl and refrigerate to marinate overnight.
In a big pot or Dutch oven, heat vegetable oil over medium-high heat. Cook and mix ginger, garlic, and onions for about 10 minutes, till golden brown. Put in the pork marinade and the pork, and cook for approximately 5 minutes, mixing often, till cubes of

pork have firmed. Add water, simmer, then lower the heat, place on the cover, and cook for about 40 minutes till pork is soft.

Mix in a quarter cup of vinegar and strips of green chile pepper. Cook without a cover for an additional of half an hour till vindaloo thickens and green chile peppers softens. Season with salt to taste prior to serving.

GOAN PRAWN PULAO

Serv.: 6| **Prep.:** 10m | **Cook:** 20m

Ingredients:
- ✓ 1/2 pound prawns, peeled and deveined
- ✓ Sea salt to taste
- ✓ 1/2 cup grated coconut
- ✓ 4 Kashmiri chile peppers
- ✓ 1 tablespoon coriander seeds
- ✓ 3 cloves garlic, peeled
- ✓ 5 peppercorns
- ✓ 1 tablespoon vegetable oil
- ✓ 1 small onion, sliced
- ✓ 1/4 teaspoon ground turmeric
- ✓ 1 1/2 cups water, or as needed
- ✓ 3 ounces okra, cut into thirds
- ✓ 3 pieces kokum

Directions: Season prawns with sea salt.

Using a mortar and pestle to crush peppercorns, garlic, coriander seeds, chile peppers, and coconut together until the masala is evenly orange.

In a pot, heat oil over medium heat, stir and cook the onion for 5-10 minutes until slightly browned and tender. Stir turmeric and masala into the onion, cook for 1 minute until aromatic. Fill with enough water to create a creamy and substantial gravy.

Boil the gravy, add okra and prawns and cook for 10 minutes until the okra is soft and the prawns are heated through. Mix kokum in the prawn mixture and boil again. Take the pot away from the heat and let sit.

GOAT AND BUTTERNUT SQUASH STEW

Serv.: 4| **Prep.:** 15m | **Cook:** 1h50m

Ingredients:
- ✓ 1 teaspoon ground cumin
- ✓ 1 teaspoon ground coriander
- ✓ 1 teaspoon ground ginger
- ✓ 1/2 teaspoon sweet paprika
- ✓ 1/2 teaspoon smoked sweet paprika
- ✓ 1/2 teaspoon smoked hot paprika
- ✓ 1/2 teaspoon ancho chile powder
- ✓ 1 (3 pound) bone-in goat shank
- ✓ 1/4 teaspoon salt, or more to taste
- ✓ 1/4 teaspoon ground black pepper, or to taste
- ✓ 2 tablespoons coconut oil
- ✓ 1 onion, chopped
- ✓ 1 (1 pound) butternut squash, peeled and cut into 1/2-inch cubes
- ✓ 4 cloves garlic, minced
- ✓ 1 (14 ounce) can diced tomatoes
- ✓ 1 1/2 cups water
- ✓ 1 cinnamon stick
- ✓ 1 pinch saffron

Directions: In a bowl, mix coriander, cumin, sweet paprika, ginger, smoked sweet paprika, chile powder and smoked hot paprika together.

Use about 1/4 teaspoon of pepper and 1/4 teaspoon of salt to rub goat shank.

In a large Dutch oven, heat coconut oil over medium-high heat until shimmering and melted. Cook goat shank in hot oil for around 2 to 3 minutes per side till browned as completely as you can get it. In a bowl, place shank, reserving oil in the skillet.

Set the heat of the skillet down to low heat. In the retained oil, cook and stir onion for approximately 7 to 10 minutes until softened. Add garlic and butternut squash; cook and stir for nearly 1 minute until the garlic is fragrant. Use the cumin mixture to sprinkle over the squash mixture; cook and stir for another 1 minute.

Into the squash mixture, mix water, tomatoes, saffron and cinnamon stick; place goat shank back to the Dutch oven, set the liquid to a simmer, and cook for about 90 minutes to 2 hours until the goat meat is falling from the bone and tender.

Take away shank from the Dutch oven then place to a cutting board. Strip meat from the bone and cut into pieces of bite-size. Discard bone. Blend meat into the squash mixture, add pepper and salt for seasoning, and cook for around 5 minutes until the meat is reheated.

GREEN SMOOTHIE

Serv.: 4| **Prep.:** 10m | **Cook:** 0

Ingredients:
- ✓ 2 cups water
- ✓ 1 head romaine lettuce, chopped
- ✓ 1/2 cucumber, diced
- ✓ 1 avocado, peeled and pitted
- ✓ 2 stalks celery
- ✓ 2 ounces baby spinach leaves
- ✓ Lemon, juiced
- ✓ 2 cups ice
- ✓ 1 apple, cored
- ✓ 1 banana

Directions: In a blender, blend together spinach, water, lemon juice, romaine lettuce, avocado, cucumber and celery on high for about 30 seconds until smooth. Pour banana, apple and ice into the blender and then blend for about 30 seconds until smooth.

KOSHER DILLS

Serv.: 9| **Prep.:** 15m | **Cook:** 20m

Ingredients:
- ✓ 3 cups water
- ✓ 1 cup distilled white vinegar
- ✓ 1/4 cup salt
- ✓ 2 cloves garlic, or more to taste
- ✓ 2 sprigs fresh dill, or more to taste
- ✓ 3 small cucumbers, or to taste
- ✓ 3 (1 pint) canning jars with lids and rings, or as needed

Directions: Boil salt, vinegar and water in a saucepan; cook for 2-3 minutes till salt melts. Sterilize the lids and jars for at least 5 minutes in boiling water. Pack garlic, dill and cucumbers in sterilized, hot jars. Put vinegar mixture over; fill to

within 1/4-in. from the top. Run a thin spatula/knife to remove any air bubbles around jar's insides after filling them. Use a moist paper towel to wipe the jar rims to remove any food residue. Put lids over; screw on rings.
Put a rack on the bottom of a big stockpot; use water to fill halfway. Boil; use a holder to lower the jars in boiling water, leave a 2-in. space between the jars. If needed, add more boiling water so water level is at least 1-in. above jar tops; put water on a rolling boil and cover the pot. Process for 15 minutes.
Take the jars from the stockpot; put on a wood/cloth-covered surface till cool, a few inches apart. Use a finger to press top of every lid when cool to be sure the seal is tight and lid doesn't move down or up at all; keep for 1 month minimum in a dark, cool area.

MEAT SAUCE

Serv.: 12| **Prep.:** 15m | **Cook:** 2h45m

Ingredients:
- ✓ 1 tablespoon olive oil
- ✓ 1 pound sweet Italian sausage, sliced
- ✓ 1 pound round steak, cubed
- ✓ 1 pound veal, cubed
- ✓ 4 cloves garlic, chopped
- ✓ 2 (28 ounce) cans whole peeled tomatoes, crushed
- ✓ 1 tablespoon Italian seasoning
- ✓ 1 bay leaf
- ✓ 1/2 teaspoon garlic powder
- ✓ 1/2 teaspoon dried oregano
- ✓ 1/2 teaspoon ground black pepper
- ✓ 1/2 teaspoon dried parsley
- ✓ 1 (28 ounce) can tomato sauce

Directions: Heat olive oil in skillet on medium heat; cook veal, round steak and sausage till evenly browned for 10 minutes. Take meat from skillet; drain. Keep 1 tablespoon drippings. Mix garlic into skillet with reserved meat drippings; cook on medium heat for 3 minutes. Put crushed tomatoes in skillet; season with parsley, pepper, oregano, garlic powder, bay leaf and Italian seasoning. Cook for 15 minutes. Mix tomato sauce into skillet; cook for 15 minutes. Put meat in skillet. Lower heat to low; simmer for 2 hours, occasionally mixing.

GRAPEFRUIT SMOOTHIE

Serv.: 2| **Prep.:** 10m | **Cook:** 0

Ingredients:
- ✓ 3 grapefruit, peeled and sectioned
- ✓ 1 cup cold water
- ✓ 3 ounces fresh spinach
- ✓ 6 ice cubes
- ✓ 1 (1/2 inch) piece peeled fresh ginger
- ✓ 1 teaspoon flax seeds

Directions: Blend the ice cubes, flax seeds, water, grapefruit, ginger, and spinach in a blender or NutriBullet®, until the mixture is smooth.

GREEN DRAGON VEGGIE JUICE

Serv.: 1| **Prep.:** 5m | **Cook:** 0

Ingredients:
- ✓ 1/4 large lemon
- ✓ 1 cup fresh spinach, or to taste
- ✓ 2 sprigs fresh parsley, or more to taste
- ✓ 2 stalks celery
- ✓ 1/3 small jalapeno pepper (optional)
- ✓ 1 tomato, quartered
- ✓ 1 pinch salt
- ✓ 1 cup ice, or as desired

Directions: Process through a juicer with lemon, spinach, parsley, celery, jalapeno pepper and tomato, respectively. Season the juice with salt. Fill ice to a glass and pour juice into.

GREEN SLIME SMOOTHIE

Serv.: 4| **Prep.:** 5m | **Cook:** 0

Ingredients:
- ✓ 2 cups spinach
- ✓ 2 cups frozen strawberries
- ✓ 1 banana

- ✓ 2 tablespoons honey
- ✓ 1/2 cup ice

Directions: Freeze spinach for at least 1 hour until frozen. In a blender, mix ice, spinach, honey, strawberries, and banana together and blend until smooth. Serve immediately.

GREEN TOMATO AND BELL PEPPER DELIGHT

Serv.: 6| **Prep.:** 5m | **Cook:** 10m

Ingredients:
- ✓ 2 tablespoons olive oil
- ✓ 4 green tomatoes, chopped
- ✓ 1 green bell pepper, chopped
- ✓ 2 celery, chopped
- ✓ 1 bunch green onions, chopped
- ✓ 2 tablespoons apple cider vinegar

Directions: In a big skillet, heat the olive oil on medium heat. Stir in apple cider vinegar, green onions, celery, bell pepper and green tomatoes. Sauté for around 5-10 minutes until it becomes tender-crisp.

GRILLED AUBERGINES WITH PROSCIUTTO

Serv.: 2| **Prep.:** 10m | **Cook:** 7m

Ingredients:
- ✓ 1 eggplant, ends trimmed
- ✓ 1 red bell pepper, cut into rings and seeds removed
- ✓ 1 cup spinach leaves, torn into pieces
- ✓ 1 (1/2 ounce) slice thinly sliced prosciutto di Parma
- ✓ 1 teaspoon sun-dried tomato paste
- ✓ 1 tablespoon extra virgin olive oil
- ✓ 1 tablespoon balsamic vinegar
- ✓ 1/4 teaspoon dried oregano
- ✓ Freshly ground rock salt to taste

Directions: Set the oven's broiler to preheat to 200°C (400°F).

Place red bell pepper and eggplant slices on a baking tray. Broil for around 7 minutes for them to soften.

While waiting for the eggplant and pepper, add spinach to a serving plate and drizzle balsamic vinegar and olive oil over. Dust with salt for seasoning. When the vegetables are softened, place the red bell peppers over the spinach. Spread each eggplant slice with a small amount of sun-dried tomato paste. Add a slice of prosciutto on top. Place the eggplant slices on top of peppers to create an overlapping spiral pattern. Serve right away.

GRILLED BACON STUFFED STRAWBERRIES

Serv.: 10| **Prep.:** 5m | **Cook:** 5m

Ingredients:
- ✓ 10 fresh strawberries, hulled
- ✓ 4 slices cooked bacon, chopped

Directions: Preheat the grill to medium heat and grease the grill grate with a little bit of oil.

Use a paring knife to cut a small cone-shaped hollow at the top of each of the strawberries.

Fill the hollow part of each strawberry with chopped bacon.

Put the bacon-filled strawberries on the preheated grill and let it cook for 2 minutes until it is hot, turn it often to evenly cook all sides.

GRILLED BEEF TENDERLOIN

Serv.: 13| **Prep.:** 30m | **Cook:** 55m

Ingredients:
- ✓ 1 (5 pound) whole beef tenderloin
- ✓ 6 tablespoons olive oil
- ✓ 8 large garlic cloves, minced
- ✓ 2 tablespoons minced fresh rosemary
- ✓ 1 tablespoon dried thyme leaves
- ✓ 2 tablespoons coarsely ground black pepper

- ✓ 1 tablespoon salt

Directions: To prepare the beef: Use a sharp knife to remove excess fat. For the thin tip end, fold under to about the thickness of the rest of the roast. Use butcher's twine to bind and continue to tie the roast with the twine every 1 1/2-2-in. (this can help the roast maintain its shape). Use scissors to snip the silver skin to make sure the roast does not bow while cooking. Combine salt, pepper, thyme, rosemary, garlic, and oil; rub this mixture over the roast until coated. Put the meat aside.

Set all gas burners on high for 10 minutes or build a charcoal fire in half the grill. Use tongs to lubricate the grate with a rag soaked with oil. On the hot rack, arrange the beef and grill, covered, for about 5 minutes until thoroughly seared. Flip the meat and grill, covered, for another 5 minutes until the second side has thoroughly seared.

Transfer the meat to the cool side of the charcoal grill, or turn off the burner directly beneath the meat and set the other 1 or 2 burners (depending on the grill style) to medium. Cook for 45-60 minutes until a meat thermometer reaches 130° for rosy pink when you insert one into the thickest part, depending on the grill and the size of the tenderloin. Allow the meat to sit for 15 minutes before carving.

GRILLED BEETS IN ROSEMARY VINEGAR

Serv.: 6| **Prep.:** 10m | **Cook:** 30m

Ingredients:
- ✓ 1/3 cup balsamic vinegar
- ✓ 1 teaspoon chopped fresh rosemary
- ✓ 1 clove garlic, peeled and crushed
- ✓ 1/2 teaspoon herbes de Provence
- ✓ 3 medium beets, sliced into rounds

Directions: Mix herbes de Provence, garlic, rosemary and balsamic vinegar in a medium bowl. Add beets in the mixture. Marinate for 20 minutes minimum.

Preheat outdoor grill to high heat; oil the grate lightly.

On a piece of foil, big enough to wrap all the ingredients, put the marinated mixture and beets; tightly seal. Put foil packet on the prepared grill. Cook till beets are tender for 25 minutes.
Take beets out of the packet. Put it on the grill grate directly for 2-5 minutes. Serve while hot.

GRILLED PORTOBELLO MUSHROOMS

Serv.: 3| **Prep.:** 10m | **Cook:** 10m

Ingredients:
- ✓ 3 portobello mushrooms
- ✓ 1/4 cup canola oil
- ✓ 3 tablespoons chopped onion
- ✓ 4 cloves garlic, minced
- ✓ 4 tablespoons balsamic vinegar

Directions: Clean mushrooms. Remove stems. Put aside for other use. On a plate, put caps, gill side up.
Mix vinegar, garlic, onion and oil in a small bowl. Evenly pour mixture on mushroom caps. Let it stand for an hour.
Grill for 10 minutes over hot grill. Immediately serve.

GRILLED SALMON WITH CURRIED PEACH SAUCE

Serv.: 2| **Prep.:** 15m | **Cook:** 15m

Ingredients:
- ✓ 2 fresh peaches, peeled and diced
- ✓ 1/4 cup honey
- ✓ 1 teaspoon curry powder
- ✓ Salt and pepper to taste
- ✓ 2 salmon steaks

Directions: Preheat the outdoor grill over medium-high heat and the coat grate lightly with oil.
Over medium heat, mix together the curry powder, honey, and peaches in a small saucepan. Heat to a simmer and then cook for about 10 minutes until the sauce becomes thick and peaches have broken down. Add pepper and salt to taste.

Season salmon steaks with pepper and salt and then cook for about 5 to 10 minutes on each side, depends on the thickness of the steaks, on the grill until fish easily flakes with a fork. Spread peach sauce atop salmon and serve.

GRILLED SAUSAGE STUFFED CALAMARI

Serv.: 8| **Prep.:** 20m | **Cook:** 15m

Ingredients:
- ✓ 2 tablespoons olive oil, divided, or as needed
- ✓ 1/2 cup diced onion
- ✓ 1/2 cup diced red bell pepper
- ✓ Salt and ground black pepper to taste
- ✓ 6 ounces spicy Italian sausage, removed from casings and crumbled
- ✓ 4 ounces calamari tentacles, minced
- ✓ 1/4 cup chopped fresh flat-leaf parsley
- ✓ 1 large egg
- ✓ 1/8 teaspoon smoked paprika
- ✓ 1 1/2 pounds cleaned calamari tubes
- ✓ 18 toothpicks, or as needed

Directions: In a skillet, heat 1 tablespoon olive oil on medium heat. Sauté red pepper and onion with a bit of salt in hot oil for 5-7 minutes until onion is translucent and soft. Take off heat. Cool to room temperature.
In a bowl, mix pepper, salt, smoked paprika, egg, parsley, onion mixture, minced tentacles, and sausage until evenly mixed. Place mixture in a piping bag.
Pipe the sausage mixture to tubes. Fill each tube to 2/3 full. On the top of every tube, thread a toothpick to fasten opening together. Put stuffed tubes onto a plate. Use plastic wrap to cover plate. Keep in fridge for about 1 hour to chill completely.
Heat an outdoor grill to medium-high heat. Oil grate lightly.
Brush leftover olive oil on tubes to coat all the sides. Season using salt.
On preheated grill, cook stuffed calamari for 10-12 minutes, occasionally turning, until stuffing is cooked through. An instant-read thermometer poked in the middle will say 68°C/155°F.

HAWKEYE PORK ROAST

Serv.: 10| Prep.: 5m | Cook: 1h30m

Ingredients:
- ✓ 1 (3 pound) boneless pork loin
- ✓ 2 tablespoons onion powder
- ✓ 2 tablespoons garlic powder
- ✓ 1 tablespoon ground black pepper

Directions: Turn the oven to 350°F (175°C) to preheat.
Use black pepper, garlic powder and onion powder to evenly season the pork loin; put in a roasting pan.
Cook for 90 minutes until the middle of the pork is not pink anymore. An instant-read thermometer should display 145°F (63°C) when you insert it into the middle.

HEALTHIER BAKED SLOW COOKER CHICKEN

Serv.: 6| Prep.: 25m | Cook: 8-10h

Ingredients:
- ✓ 1 (2 to 3 pound) whole chicken
- ✓ Salt and ground black pepper to taste
- ✓ 1 teaspoon paprika
- ✓ 3 large carrots, split lengthwise and cut into 2-inch pieces
- ✓ 2 medium onions, quartered
- ✓ 2 tablespoons fresh chopped parsley

Directions: Wad a piece of aluminum foil into 3- to 4-in. ball, working in the same manner to make 3 pieces; arrange them on the bottom of a slow cooker.
Rinse chicken under cold water, inside and out. Use paper towels to pat dry. Season paprika, pepper and salt on the chicken. Put the chicken into a slow cooker, on top of the crumbled aluminum foil.
Set the slow cooker on high for 1 hour; decrease to low for 4-5 hours. Add in vegetables; cook for around another 4-5 hours, or till the juices run

clear and the chicken is not pink anymore. Sprinkle parsley over. Serve.

HEALTHIER MARINATED GRILLED SHRIMP

Serv.: 6| Prep.: 15m | Cook: 6m

Ingredients:
- ✓ 3 cloves garlic, minced
- ✓ 2 tablespoons olive oil
- ✓ 1/4 cup tomato sauce
- ✓ 2 tablespoons red wine vinegar
- ✓ 2 tablespoons chopped fresh basil
- ✓ 1/2 teaspoon salt
- ✓ 1/4 teaspoon cayenne pepper
- ✓ 2 pounds fresh shrimp, peeled and deveined
- ✓ Skewers

Directions: In a large bowl, combine red wine vinegar, tomato sauce, olive oil and garlic. Use cayenne pepper, salt and basil for seasoning. Stir in shrimps until they are evenly coated. Put it in the refrigerator with cover, stirring one or two time, in 30 minutes or 1 hour.
Grease the grate lightly with oil; preheat the grill on medium heat.
Thread shrimps onto skewers, piercing once near head and once near tail. Throw away the marinate.
Put the shrimps on the preheated grill and cook for 2 to 3 minutes per side until they turns opaque.

HEALTHIER TACO SEASONING

Serv.: 10| Prep.: 5m | Cook: 0

Ingredients:
- ✓ 1 clove garlic, peeled
- ✓ 1 teaspoon sea salt
- ✓ 1 tablespoon chili powder
- ✓ 1/4 teaspoon red pepper flakes
- ✓ 1/4 teaspoon dried oregano
- ✓ 1/2 teaspoon paprika
- ✓ 1 1/2 teaspoons ground cumin
- ✓ 1 teaspoon ground black pepper

Directions: Crush the garlic with salt until it forms

into a paste. In a small bowl, stir in pepper, cumin, paprika, oregano, red pepper flakes and chili powder. On the other hand, in a bowl of a mini food processor, mix together all the ingredients until well combined. Store it in the fridge in an airtight container.

HEALTHY LAMB MEATBALLS

Serv.: 4| **Prep.:** 20m | **Cook:** 30m

Ingredients:
- ✓ 1 pound ground lamb, or more to taste
- ✓ 1/2 cup shredded cabbage, or more to taste
- ✓ 1/3 cup diced onion
- ✓ 1 egg
- ✓ 1 1/4 tablespoons ground allspice
- ✓ 1 tablespoon freshly ground cardamom
- ✓ 1/4 teaspoon ground turmeric (optional)
- ✓ 1/4 teaspoon ground sumac (optional)
- ✓ Salt and ground black pepper to taste

Directions: Start preheating the oven at 350°F (175°C).
In a pot of water, heat lamb to a boil, crumbling into small chunks, using a spoon, until cooked completely, for 5 to 10 minutes. Discard fat from the water by a spoon and drain water from meat. Combine pepper, salt, sumac, turmeric, cardamom, allspice, egg, onion, cabbage, and cooked lamb in a bowl; roll to form into 1 1/2-inch balls.
Put meatballs on a baking sheet.
Bake in the prepared oven until meatballs are cooked thoroughly and turn brown on the outside, for 25 to 30 minutes.

HEARTY VENISON AND VEGETABLE BAKE

Serv.: 4| **Prep.:** 20m | **Cook:** 50m

Ingredients:
- ✓ 1 pound venison, cut into cubes
- ✓ 1 pound mushrooms, quartered
- ✓ 4 green onions, cut into 1/2-inch pieces
- ✓ 1 bulb fennel, sliced
- ✓ 2 parsnips, peeled and cut into 1/2 inch slices
- ✓ 2 tablespoons olive oil
- ✓ Salt and pepper to taste

Directions: Preheat an oven to 175 °C or 350 °F.
In olive oil, toss parsnips, fennel, green onion, mushrooms and venison. Season with pepper and salt to taste; coat by tossing. Place onto a glass baking dish.
In prepped oven, bake for approximately 50 minutes till venison and vegetables are soft and browned.

HUNGARIAN GOULASH

Serv.: 8| **Prep.:** 15m | **Cook:** 2h

Ingredients:
- ✓ 1/3 cup vegetable oil
- ✓ 3 onions, sliced
- ✓ 2 tablespoons Hungarian sweet paprika
- ✓ 2 teaspoons salt
- ✓ 1/2 teaspoon ground black pepper
- ✓ 3 pounds beef stew meat, cut into 1 1/2 inch cubes
- ✓ 1 (6 ounce) can tomato paste
- ✓ 1 1/2 cups water
- ✓ 1 clove garlic, minced
- ✓ 1 teaspoon salt

Directions: On medium heat, heat oil in a Dutch oven or big pot; add onions. Cook and stir frequently until soft. Take out onions and let it stand.
Mix together pepper, 2 teaspoons of salt, and paprika in a medium bowl. Dredge beef cubes in the mixture. Cook beef cubes in the onion pot until all sides are brown. Place the onions back in the pot; add leftover a teaspoon of salt, tomato paste, garlic, and water. Turn heat to low and let it simmer, covered for 1 1/2 - 2 hrs until the beef is tender; stir from time to time.

HUNGARIAN HOT AND SPICY PICKLED CAULIFLOWER

Serv.: 39| **Prep.:** 20m | **Cook:** 10m

Ingredients:
- ✓ 4 cups distilled white vinegar
- ✓ 4 cups water
- ✓ 1/2 cup sea salt
- ✓ 1 head cauliflower, broken into florets
- ✓ 3 hot chile peppers, sliced lengthwise
- ✓ 3 cloves garlic, minced, divided
- ✓ 1 tablespoon mustard seed, divided
- ✓ 1 tablespoon whole black peppercorns, divided
- ✓ 1 tablespoon coriander seeds, divided
- ✓ 1 tablespoon dill seeds, divided
- ✓ 1 tablespoon allspice berries, divided
- ✓ 1 1/2 teaspoons red pepper flakes, divided
- ✓ 3 bay leaves
- ✓ 3 1-quart canning jars with lids and rings

Directions: In pot, mix salt, water and vinegar together; simmer.

In boiling water, sterilize lids and jars for a minimum of 5 minutes. Fill each jar with 1 bay leaf, half teaspoon red pepper flakes, a teaspoon allspice berries, a teaspoon dill seed, a teaspoon coriander seed, 1 teaspoon peppercorns, 1 teaspoon mustard seed, a minced garlic clove, a hot pepper and 1/3 cauliflower. Into jars, add vinegar mixture, filling to within half-inch of surface. Run a thin spatula or knife surrounding the inner of jars when filled to get rid of any air bubbles. Using moist paper towel, wipe jars rims to get rid of any food residue. Put lids on and screw on the rings.

In the base of a big stockpot, put a rack and fill with water midway. Boil and into boiling water, put down the jars with holder. Retain a 2 inches gap between jars. Put in additional boiling water if needed, for water level to reach at minimum of an-inch over the jar tops. Let water come to a rolling boil, put cover on pot, and process for 10 minutes. Take jars out of stockpot and put onto a wood or cloth-covered surface, a few inches away, till cool. When cool, push the surface of every lid using finger, making sure that seal is tight, lid should not move down or up at all. Keep in a dark, cool place.

HUNTER STYLE CHICKEN

Serv.: 4 | **Prep.:** 15m | **Cook:** 40m

Ingredients:
- ✓ 4 tablespoons olive oil
- ✓ 1 (3 pound) whole chicken, cut into pieces
- ✓ 6 slices bacon, diced
- ✓ 2 onions, chopped
- ✓ 1 cup fresh sliced mushrooms
- ✓ 1 tablespoon chopped fresh parsley
- ✓ 1 tablespoon chopped fresh basil
- ✓ 1 teaspoon salt
- ✓ Freshly ground black pepper
- ✓ 1 cup white wine
- ✓ 1 pound tomatoes, diced

Directions: In a large skillet, heat oil; brown the chicken; remove. Add bacon; sauté for about 2 minutes over medium heat.

Add onions and mushrooms and keep sautéing until onions become translucent. Transfer chicken back to the skillet; scatter with pepper, salt, basil and parsley. Add tomatoes and wine. Simmer, covered, for 25-30 minutes; during cooking, turning the chicken once. Take the chicken out of the skillet; pour the sauce over the chicken.

HUNTER'S BEET CHIPS

Serv.: 4 | **Prep.:** 15m | **Cook:** 30m

Ingredients:
- ✓ Cooking spray
- ✓ 5 large beets, peeled and thinly sliced
- ✓ 1 tablespoon olive oil, or as needed
- ✓ Salt and ground black pepper to taste

Directions: Prepare oven by heating it to 200° C or 400° F. Use cooking spray to grease a baking sheet. Arrange beets in one layer on the prepared baking sheet. Brush with olive oil on both sides of the beets. Add pepper and salt to taste.

Bake in oven for 15 minutes. Flip beets and cook for 15-20 minutes more until crisp. Move to wire rack and cool.

HURRICANE CARROTS

Serv.: 6| **Prep.:** 10m | **Cook:** 0

Ingredients:
- ✓ 1 cup shredded carrots
- ✓ 1 cup finely chopped apple
- ✓ 1/2 cup raisins
- ✓ 1/2 cup golden raisins
- ✓ 1 cup whole almonds
- ✓ 1/2 cup vegetable oil
- ✓ Salt and ground black pepper to taste

Directions: In a medium bowl, combine oil with almonds, all raisins, apple and carrots. Add pepper and salt for seasoning.

BREAKFAST SAUSAGE PATTIES

Serv.: 16| **Prep.:** 20m | **Cook:** 10m

Ingredients:
- ✓ 3 pounds ground pork
- ✓ 1 tablespoon molasses
- ✓ 1 tablespoon kosher salt
- ✓ 2 teaspoons ground black pepper, or to taste
- ✓ 1 1/2 teaspoons dried sage
- ✓ 1 1/2 teaspoons dried thyme
- ✓ 1 teaspoon red pepper flakes (optional)
- ✓ 1 teaspoon onion powder
- ✓ 1 teaspoon chopped fresh parsley
- ✓ 3/4 teaspoon ground nutmeg
- ✓ 1/2 teaspoon fennel seeds
- ✓ 1/2 teaspoon ground cayenne
- ✓ 1/2 teaspoon ground allspice

Directions: By hand, mix allspice, cayenne, fennel seeds, nutmeg, parsley, onion powder, red pepper flakes, thyme, sage, black pepper, salt, molasses and pork well in big bowl.
Divide the pork mixture to 16 portions; form into 1/4-in. thick patties.
Heat nonstick skillet on medium heat; in batches, pan-fry patties for 5 minutes per side till not pink in middle anymore and golden.

REAL MEXICAN CEVICHE

Serv.: 12| **Prep.:** 15m | **Cook:** 0

Ingredients:
- ✓ 4 pounds shrimp
- ✓ 1 pound scallops
- ✓ 6 large limes, juiced
- ✓ 1 large lemon, juiced
- ✓ 1 small white onion, chopped
- ✓ 1 cucumber, peeled and chopped
- ✓ 1 large tomato, coarsely chopped
- ✓ 1 jalapeno pepper, chopped
- ✓ 1 serrano pepper, chopped
- ✓ 1 bunch cilantro
- ✓ 1 tablespoon olive oil
- ✓ 1 tablespoon kosher salt
- ✓ Ground black pepper to taste

Directions: Toss the scallops and shrimp gently in a ceramic bowl or big glass with lemon juice and lime juice. Combine the pepper, salt, olive oil, cilantro, serrano, jalapeno, tomato, cucumber and onion. Cover the bowl and let the ceviche chill for an hour in the fridge, until the scallops and shrimp become opaque.

PORK CHORIZO

Serv.: 6| **Prep.:** 15m | **Cook:** 0

Ingredients:
- ✓ 2 pounds ground pork
- ✓ 2 teaspoons salt
- ✓ 4 tablespoons chili powder
- ✓ 1/4 teaspoon ground cloves
- ✓ 2 tablespoons paprika
- ✓ 2 cloves garlic, crushed
- ✓ 1 teaspoon dried oregano
- ✓ 3 1/2 tablespoons cider vinegar

Directions: Combine vinegar, oregano, garlic, paprika, ground cloves, chili powder, salt, and ground pork well. Put in an air-tight container to store in the fridge for the spices to combine before using, about 4 days.

JUMPING GINGER SMOOTHIE

Serv.: 1| **Prep.:** 15m | **Cook:** 0

Ingredients:
- ✓ 2 cups cold water
- ✓ 1 avocado, peeled, and pitted
- ✓ 1/2 cup fresh parsley
- ✓ 1 apple, cored and seeded
- ✓ 1 carrot, cut into chunks
- ✓ 1 lemon, peeled
- ✓ 1 leaf kale leaf, or more to taste
- ✓ 1 (1 inch) piece fresh ginger root, or more to taste
- ✓ 2 ice cubes (optional)
- ✓ 1 tablespoon flax seeds (optional)

Directions: Blend flax seeds, kale, apple, avocado, ice cubes, parsley, water, carrot, ginger, and lemon in a blender at high speed for 10-15 seconds until the mixture is smooth.

JUST PLAIN OL' CHILI

Serv.: 6| **Prep.:** 15m | **Cook:** 2h45m

Ingredients:
- ✓ 2 pounds lean ground beef
- ✓ 2 tablespoons olive oil
- ✓ 1 green bell pepper, diced
- ✓ 6 cloves garlic, minced
- ✓ 3 tablespoons ground cumin
- ✓ 1 tablespoon chili powder, or more to taste
- ✓ Salt and ground black pepper to taste
- ✓ 1 (28 ounce) can diced tomatoes
- ✓ 4 cups water

Directions: In a large skillet, heat over medium heat and add the ground beef; cook and stir until meat is not pink anymore, evenly browned, and crumbled, about 10 minutes. Discard all the excess grease.
Heat olive oil on medium-high heat in a soup pot. Cook and stir green pepper in the hot oil until it begins to soften, about 5 to 7 minutes. Lower the heat to low, blend in chili powder, cumin, and

garlic, and flavor with salt and black pepper to taste.
Combine cooked ground beef and tomatoes in the green bell pepper mixture, using a spatula to crumble tomatoes. Pour in 4 cups of water, or until enough to cover the ingredients, lower the heat to low, and simmer for at least 2 hours for the flavors to be well-blended.

KADHAI MURGH WITH BELL PEPPER

Serv.: 6| **Prep.:** 15m | **Cook:** 45m

Ingredients:
- ✓ 1 1/2 pounds skinless, boneless chicken breast, cut into bite-sized chunks
- ✓ 1/2 teaspoon salt
- ✓ 1/2 teaspoon ground turmeric
- ✓ 1/4 cup vegetable oil
- ✓ 2 onions, sliced thin
- ✓ 2 green bell peppers, cut into thin strips
- ✓ 4 green chile peppers, halved lengthwise
- ✓ 1/2 teaspoon cumin seed
- ✓ 1/2 teaspoon coriander seed
- ✓ 1/2 teaspoon whole black peppercorns
- ✓ 1/2 cinnamon stick
- ✓ 6 whole cloves
- ✓ 1 black cardamom pod
- ✓ 1/4 teaspoon fennel seed
- ✓ 1/2 cup water
- ✓ 2 tablespoons coconut milk powder
- ✓ 1/2 teaspoon ground red pepper
- ✓ Salt to taste
- ✓ 1/4 cup chopped fresh cilantro

Directions: Season the chicken evenly with turmeric and salt; put aside for 15 minutes.
In a kadhai or big skillet, heat oil over medium heat. In hot oil, let the onions cook for about 5 minutes till browned. Put in chicken and cook for an additional of approximately 5 minutes till browned. Into the chicken, mix chile peppers and bell peppers; keep cooking for 5 minutes more. Grind fennel seed, cardamom pod, cloves, cinnamon, black peppercorns, coriander seed and cumin seed into a coarse powder; scatter on top of mixture in the skillet. Put in salt, ground red

pepper, coconut milk powder and water. Cook for about half an hour till chicken is soft. Incase curry is too wet, cook on high till moisture evaporates. Jazz up with cilantro and serve while hot.

KALE CHIPS

Serv.: 2| **Prep.:** 15m | **Cook:** 35m

Ingredients:
- ✓ 1 bunch kale
- ✓ 1 tablespoon extra-virgin olive oil, divided
- ✓ 1 tablespoon sherry vinegar
- ✓ 1 pinch sea salt, to taste

Directions: Prepare oven by heating to 150° C or 300° F.
Remove inner ribs of each kale leaf and throw away. Tear the leaves evenly to pieces. (Usually about a size of a small potato chip when I make it.) Wash the leaves then dry using a salad spinner or with paper towels to completely remove water. Place kale pieces in a big resealable bag or a bowl if you want to use your hands. Place about half of the olive oil. Seal the bag and squeeze it so the oil coats kale evenly. Add the rest of the oil and squeeze the bag some more. Slightly "massage", making sure the oil evenly coats the leaves. Add the vinegar on kale leaves, seal the bag again, and shake to evenly distribute the vinegar on all the leaves. Arrange the leaves on a baking sheet evenly.
Roast in the oven for 35 minutes until almost crisp. Add salt to taste. Immediately serve.

PALEO ZUCCHINI CHIPS

Serv.: 6| **Prep.:** 15m | **Cook:** 45m

Ingredients:
- ✓ 1 tablespoon grated lime zest
- ✓ 2 teaspoons lime juice
- ✓ 2 teaspoons smoked paprika
- ✓ 1 teaspoon kosher salt
- ✓ 1/2 teaspoon ground black pepper
- ✓ 2 large zucchinis, thinly sliced
- ✓ Cooking spray

Directions: Heat oven to 110 degrees Celsius or 225 degrees Fahrenheit. Place parchment paper on a baking sheet.
Mix pepper, salt, paprika, lime juice, and lime zest in a bowl.
Put zucchini slices in one layer on the baking sheet. Grease using cooking spray then sprinkle lime mix on the top.
Bake in oven for 45-60 minutes until crispy and golden.

KOFTA KEBABS

Serv.: 28| **Prep.:** 45m | **Cook:** 5m

Ingredients:
- ✓ 4 cloves garlic, minced
- ✓ 1 teaspoon kosher salt
- ✓ 1 pound ground lamb
- ✓ 3 tablespoons grated onion
- ✓ 3 tablespoons chopped fresh parsley
- ✓ 1 tablespoon ground coriander
- ✓ 1 teaspoon ground cumin
- ✓ 1/2 tablespoon ground cinnamon
- ✓ 1/2 teaspoon ground allspice
- ✓ 1/4 teaspoon cayenne pepper
- ✓ 1/4 teaspoon ground ginger
- ✓ 1/4 teaspoon ground black pepper
- ✓ 28 bamboo skewers, soaked in water for 30 minutes

Directions: Use a mortar and pestle to mash garlic with salt until paste like. Use the flat side of the chef's knife and chopping board as an alternative way to create the paste. Stir garlic, onion, coriander, cumin, parsley, allspice, ginger, cayenne pepper, cinnamon, and pepper with lamb in a bowl. Stir mixture until well incorporated then mold in 28 balls. Make every ball around the tip of skewer and flat each into a 2-inch oval. Repeat with the rest of the skewers. On a baking sheet and transfer kebabs. For 30 minutes to 12 hours, refrigerate with cover.
Prepare the grill by lightly oiling the grate and preheat at medium heat.

Place the skewers on heated grill. Grill lamb while flipping occasionally until cooked to your desired doneness. For medium, grill 6 minutes.

KOREAN CUCUMBER SALAD

Serv.: 2| **Prep.:** 20m | **Cook:** 5m

Ingredients:
- ✓ 1/4 cup white vinegar
- ✓ 1/4 teaspoon black pepper
- ✓ 1/2 teaspoon red pepper flakes
- ✓ 1 teaspoon vegetable oil
- ✓ 2 tablespoons sesame seeds
- ✓ 1 cucumber, thinly sliced
- ✓ 1/2 green onion, sliced
- ✓ 1/2 carrot, julienned

Directions: Mix red pepper flakes, black pepper, and vinegar in a medium bowl.
In a saucepan, heat oil on medium-high heat. Mix in sesame seeds. Reduce the heat to medium. Cook for 5 minutes until seeds become brown. Take seeds out using a slotted spoon. Mix into the vinegar mixture. Stir in carrot, green onions, and cucumber. Cover then keep in fridge for at least five minutes.

SWEET POTATO FRIES

Serv.: 4| **Prep.:** 30m | **Cook:** 20m

Ingredients:
- ✓ 4 sweet potatoes, peeled and cut into long French fries
- ✓ 1/4 cup olive oil
- ✓ 1 teaspoon steak seasoning
- ✓ 1/2 teaspoon ground black pepper
- ✓ 1/2 teaspoon garlic powder
- ✓ 1/4 teaspoon salt
- ✓ 1/4 teaspoon paprika
- ✓ 1 tablespoon olive oil

Directions: In a big bowl, put sweet potato fries, sprinkle with a quarter cup olive oil, and coat by tossing. In another small bowl, combine paprika, salt, garlic powder, black pepper and steak seasoning till well mixed. Toss fries with olive oil using your left hand while drizzle the seasoning mixture over using right hand.
In a big skillet over medium heat, heat a tablespoon olive oil and put sweet potato pieces into the hot oil. Cover skillet and, pan-fry for 5 minutes; remove cover and flip fries. Put back cover over fries and cook for additional 5 minutes; keep flipping fries and covering for 10 minutes longer till sweet potatoes are soft.

LA GENOVESE

Serv.: 6| **Prep.:** 5m | **Cook:** 10m

Ingredients:
- ✓ 1/2 cup olive oil
- ✓ 1 pound lean ground beef
- ✓ 3 carrots, diced
- ✓ 1/2 onion, minced
- ✓ 1 teaspoon salt
- ✓ 1 pinch ground black pepper
- ✓ 3 tablespoons white wine

Directions: Put a large skillet over medium heat to heat olive oil. Add in beef; cook and stir well to break up clumps until it starts to brown. Add pepper, salt, onion and carrots; stir well. Cook for another 5 minutes with stirs until the meat extracts clear juice and the vegetables are just tender. Put in wine; continue cooking for another 1 minute and serve.

MANGO SALSA ON TILAPIA FILLETS

Serv.: 4| **Prep.:** 30m | **Cook:** 10m

Ingredients:
- ✓ 1/2 fresh pineapple - peeled, cored, and chopped
- ✓ 1/2 pound strawberries, quartered
- ✓ 3 kiwifruit, peeled and diced
- ✓ 1 large mango - peeled, seeded and diced
- ✓ 1/2 cup grape tomatoes
- ✓ 2 tablespoons finely chopped fresh cilantro
- ✓ 1 tablespoon balsamic vinegar
- ✓ 1 1/2 pounds tilapia fillets
- ✓ 1/2 teaspoon seasoned pepper blend

Directions: Add strawberries, mango, cilantro, tomatoes, pineapple, balsamic vinegar and kiwifruit in a bowl and toss it together.

Add a cooking spray in a pan and heat it over medium-high heat. Add seasoned pepper blend to the tilapia for seasoning and cook the fish in the frying pan for 2-3 minutes per side, until the fish turns opaque and white in color. Add the salsa on top of the fish before serving.

LAMB AND ASPARAGUS STEW

Serv.: 2| **Prep.:** 20m | **Cook:** 35m

Ingredients:
- ✓ 3 tablespoons vegetable oil
- ✓ 1 onion, chopped
- ✓ 1/2 pound cubed lamb stew meat
- ✓ 1/2 teaspoon salt
- ✓ 1/2 teaspoon ground black pepper
- ✓ 1 tablespoon ground turmeric
- ✓ 1/2 (6 ounce) can tomato paste
- ✓ 1 cup water
- ✓ 1 clove garlic, chopped
- ✓ 1 bunch fresh asparagus, trimmed and cut into 1 inch pieces

Directions: In a saucepan over medium high heat, heat vegetable oil. Stir in onions and cook for 2 minutes, remember to stir constantly while cooking. Add turmeric, pepper, salt and lamb; cook for about 3 minutes until the outside of lamb loses its pink color, remember to stir while cooking. Stir in garlic, water and tomato paste. Bring to a simmer, then lower the heat to medium-low, cover the saucepan and simmer for about 25 minutes until the lamb is softened.

When the lamb is soft, stir in asparagus and keep cooking for 3 minutes until asparagus is tender.

ROASTED SWEET POTATO BITES

Serv.: 1| **Prep.:** 10m | **Cook:** 20m

Ingredients:
- ✓ 1 cup peeled and cubed sweet potato
- ✓ 1/2 teaspoon coconut oil, melted
- ✓ 1 1/2 teaspoons chopped fresh rosemary
- ✓ 1 1/2 teaspoons chopped fresh thyme
- ✓ Salt and ground black pepper to taste

Directions: Set the oven to 190°C or 375°F.

In a bowl, add sweet potato cubes. Drizzle over potatoes with coconut oil and toss with your hands, until each cubes is coated. Spread the sweet potato cubes on a baking sheet, then season with pepper, salt, thyme and rosemary.

In the preheated oven, bake potatoes for approximately 20 minutes, until tender.

COCONUT FLAX MUG MUFFINS

Serv.: 1| **Prep.:** 5m | **Cook:** 1m

Ingredients:
- ✓ 1 egg
- ✓ 1/4 cup golden flaxseed meal
- ✓ 1 tablespoon unsweetened coconut flakes
- ✓ 1 teaspoon coconut oil
- ✓ 1 teaspoon unsweetened coconut milk beverage (such as Silk®)
- ✓ 1 teaspoon vanilla extract
- ✓ 1/2 teaspoon baking powder
- ✓ 1/2 teaspoon stevia powder

Directions: In a bowl, combine stevia, baking powder, vanilla extract, coconut beverage, coconut oil, coconut flakes, flaxseed meal and egg, then mix well. Place the batter into the microwave-safe mug. Cook for one minute on high in the microwave oven.

LOW CARB ZUCCHINI CHIPS

Serv.: 2| **Prep.:** 10m | **Cook:** 2h

Ingredients:
- ✓ 2 large large zucchini, thinly sliced
- ✓ 1 tablespoon olive oil, or to taste
- ✓ Sea salt to taste

Directions: Heat oven to 120 degrees Celsius or 250 degrees Fahrenheit.

Place the cut zucchini on the baking sheet. Lightly drizzle using olive oil and lightly sprinkle with some sea salt.

Bake in the oven for an hour on each side until they're like chips and entirely dry. Let it cool before eating.

LOW CARB ZUCCHINI PASTA

Serv.: 1| **Prep.:** 10m | **Cook:** 5m

Ingredients:
- ✓ 2 zucchinis, peeled
- ✓ 1 tablespoon olive oil
- ✓ 1/4 cup water
- ✓ Salt and ground black pepper to taste

Directions: Use a veggie peeler to cut zucchini lengthwise, stop when the seeds appear. Flip zucchini over and peel the rest of it into long strips; throw out seeds.

Slice zucchini strips into thinner threads that look like spaghetti.

In a big frying pan, heat olive oil on medium; cook the zucchini in the hot oil and stir, 1 minute. Add the water and cook 5-7 minutes until zucchini becomes soft. Use pepper and salt to season.

QUICKIE CHICKIE

Serv.: 2| **Prep.:** 10m | **Cook:** 10m

Ingredients:
- ✓ 2 teaspoons olive oil
- ✓ 6 ounces chicken tenderloin strips
- ✓ 1/4 teaspoon salt
- ✓ 1/8 teaspoon freshly ground black pepper
- ✓ 2 tablespoons chopped fresh basil
- ✓ 1 1/2 teaspoons honey
- ✓ 1 1/2 teaspoons balsamic vinegar, or more to taste

Directions: On medium-high heat, pour olive oil in a non-stick pan and heat. Sprinkle pepper and salt

on the chicken. Cook while regularly stirring the chicken in the hot oil for 3-5 minutes until it's not pink in the middle. Mix honey, balsamic vinegar, and basil into the chicken and stir Cook for another minute.

MAGARICZ

Serv.: 10| **Prep.:** 20m | **Cook:** 40m

Ingredients:
- ✓ 1/4 cup olive oil
- ✓ 1 large eggplant, peeled and coarsely chopped
- ✓ 1 medium red bell pepper, cut into thin strips
- ✓ 1 green bell pepper, cut into thin strips
- ✓ 1 large onion, diced
- ✓ 1 cup coarsely shredded carrot
- ✓ Salt to taste
- ✓ Crushed red pepper flakes

Directions: Lightly salt eggplant and place in a colander. Set aside for about 45 minutes, allowing eggplant to drain.

Heat olive oil in a big pan over medium high heat. Toss in eggplant, onion, carrot, red and green bell peppers.

Mix well to coat then turn heat down to low. Continue cooking for 40 minutes, stirring from time to time, until mixture achieves coarse jam consistency. Sprinkle with salt and red pepper flakes to taste.

Refrigerate, covered, for at least 1 hour. Serve chilled with your preferred crackers or bread.

MANGO CHUTNEY

Serv.: 32| **Prep.:** 40m | **Cook:** 35m

Ingredients:
- ✓ 4 cups green (under ripe) mangoes - peeled, seeded, and diced
- ✓ 1/2 cup raisins
- ✓ 1/4 cup serrano peppers, finely chopped
- ✓ 6 cloves garlic, minced
- ✓ 1 1/2 tablespoons minced fresh ginger root

- ✓ 1 1/2 teaspoons lemon zest
- ✓ 1 tablespoon black pepper
- ✓ 2 tablespoons molasses
- ✓ 1 small cinnamon stick
- ✓ 4 whole cloves
- ✓ 1 cup water
- ✓ 1 cup cider vinegar

Directions: In a large saucepan, place cloves, cinnamon, molasses, black pepper, lemon zest, ginger, garlic, serrano peppers, raisins and mango. Transfer in vinegar and water.
Boil the mixture; turn the heat down to medium-low and simmer without a cover for around 30 minutes, or till it reaches a jam-like consistency. Mix frequently while cooking.
Allow to cool when thickened; place in a refrigerator for storage. You can also freeze the chutney.

MAPLE GLAZED BUTTERNUT SQUASH

Serv.: 4 | **Prep.:** 10m | **Cook:** 20m

Ingredients:
- ✓ 1 butternut squash - peeled, seeded, quartered, and cut into 1/2-inch slices
- ✓ 2/3 cup water
- ✓ 1/4 cup maple syrup
- ✓ 1/4 cup dark rum
- ✓ 1/4 teaspoon ground nutmeg

Directions: Boil nutmeg, butternut squash, rum, maple syrup, and water together in a pot. Lower heat; let it simmer for 15m while stirring occasionally until the squash is tender.
With a slotted spoon move the butternut squash to a serving dish; save the liquid in the pot.
Simmer for 5-10m until the liquid is thick and reduced; pour all over the butternut squash.

MAPLE GLAZED CHICKEN WITH SWEET POTATOES

Serv.: 4 | **Prep.:** 15m | **Cook:** 30m

Ingredients:

- ✓ 1 1/2 pounds sweet potatoes, peeled and cut into 1-inch pieces
- ✓ 1 pound chicken tenders
- ✓ 2 teaspoons steak seasoning (such as Montreal Steak Seasoning®)
- ✓ 2 tablespoons vegetable oil
- ✓ 1/2 cup maple syrup
- ✓ 1/2 cup sliced green onions

Directions: Put the sweet potatoes into a large pot and add water to cover. Bring to a boil over high heat, then lower the heat to medium-low, and simmer for about 20 minutes, covered, until softened.
Drain and let them steam dry for a minute or two. Mash the potatoes and put aside.
Dust steak seasoning over chicken tenders; put oil in a large skillet and heat over medium heat, then add the chicken tenders and cook for 5-8 minutes each side, until the meat is not pink anymore inside and lightly browned.
Take off the chicken, and put aside Whisk maple syrup into the skillet, scraping up and dissolving any browned flavor bits from the skillet. Bring to a boil, simmer for 2 minutes, and mix in the green onions.
Put the mashed sweet potatoes onto a serving platter with chicken tenders on top and pour maple sauce over the chicken to serve.

MAPLE GLAZED SWEET POTATOES WITH BACON & CARAMELIZED ONIONS

Serv.: 12 | **Prep.:** 30m | **Cook:** 1h5m

Ingredients:
- ✓ 4 pounds sweet potatoes, peeled and cut in 1-inch chunks
- ✓ 2 tablespoons olive oil
- ✓ 1 teaspoon salt
- ✓ 1/2 teaspoon ground black pepper
- ✓ 5 slices smoked bacon, chopped
- ✓ 1 pound onions, thinly sliced
- ✓ 1 cup pure maple syrup
- ✓ 2 teaspoons fresh thyme

Directions: Preheat an oven to 220 °C or 425 °F. In

a big bowl, toss black pepper, salt, olive oil and sweet potato chunks. On a big rimmed baking sheet, arrange the sweet potatoes.

In the prepped oven, roast for 40 minutes till soft and browned; mix after the initial 20 minutes. In a big skillet over medium heat, cook the bacon for 10 minutes till brown and crisp; put the bacon into a bowl, but retain grease in the skillet. In bacon grease, cook onions for 10 minutes till browned, mixing often. Turn heat down to low, and cook the onions for 10 to 15 minutes more till really tender, sweet and brown. Mix frequently. Blend onions with bacon in the bowl, and reserve. In the hot skillet, put maple syrup with thyme, and bring to a rolling boil. Boil syrup for 3 to 4 minutes till reduced by half. Put in onion-bacon mixture and roasted sweet potatoes, coat vegetables with maple glaze by mixing. Place into a serving dish.

MARINATED GRILLED SHRIMP

Serv.: 6| **Prep.:** 15m | **Cook:** 6m

Ingredients:
- ✓ 3 cloves garlic, minced
- ✓ 1/3 cup olive oil
- ✓ 1/4 cup tomato sauce
- ✓ 2 tablespoons red wine vinegar
- ✓ 2 tablespoons chopped fresh basil
- ✓ 1/2 teaspoon salt
- ✓ 1/4 teaspoon cayenne pepper
- ✓ 2 pounds fresh shrimp, peeled and deveined
- ✓ Skewers

Directions: Mix together red wine vinegar, tomato sauce, olive oil, and garlic in a large bowl. Sprinkle with salt, cayenne pepper, and basil. Put in the shrimps and stir to coat. Cover and refrigerate for half up to a full hour, stirring occasionally. Preheat grill at medium. Skewer the shrimps, impaling near the tail and coming out near the head. Discard its marinade.

Lightly grease the grate. Grill for 2 to 3 minutes each side or until flesh is opaque.

MARINATED KEBABS

Serv.: 4| **Prep.:** 40m| **Cook:** 10m

Ingredients:
- ✓ 2 pounds premium meat
- ✓ 2 bell peppers (color of your choice)
- ✓ 1 onion
- ✓ 1/4 teaspoon dried thyme
- ✓ Salt and pepper
- ✓ 3 tablespoons olive oil
- ✓ 1 jar Maille® Dijon Originale Mustard
- ✓ Skewers

Directions: Slice the meat, onions, and bell peppers into squares.

Whisk together the contents of a jar of Maille® Dijon Originale mustard, thyme, olive oil, and salt and pepper in a large bowl. Toss in the meat to coat and marinate in the refrigerator for half an hour. Cue the meat alternately with the onions and the bell peppers onto skewers. Flip and baste frequently with remaining mixture while grilling.

CLAM CHOWDER

Serv.: 12| **Prep.:** 15m | **Cook:** 45m

Ingredients:
- ✓ 8 slices bacon
- ✓ 1 cup chopped onion
- ✓ 1 cup chopped celery
- ✓ 7 cups clam juice
- ✓ 3 (28 ounce) cans stewed tomatoes
- ✓ 5 tablespoons dried thyme
- ✓ 2 (6.5 ounce) cans minced clams

Directions: On medium heat, fry the bacon in a large saucepan until the meat turns crisp. Until done, remove from the pot and crush. In the same pot, cook the onion and celery until the onion turns translucent. Add in the tomatoes and clam juice. Season the mixture with thyme and then mix in the clams. Let simmer for 45 minutes for the flavors to blend well together.

MARINATED MUSHROOMS

Serv.: 8| **Prep.:** 10m | **Cook:** 0

Ingredients:
- ✓ 1 1/2 teaspoons garlic salt
- ✓ 1 1/2 teaspoons seasoning salt
- ✓ 1/4 cup distilled white vinegar
- ✓ 1/2 cup olive oil
- ✓ 2 (8 ounce) cans mushrooms, drained

Directions: Whisk the olive oil, vinegar, seasoned salt and garlic salt together. Spread over mushrooms and let marinate for 24 hours.

BAKED ONIONS

Serv.: 6| **Prep.:** 1h | **Cook:** 30m

Ingredients:
- ✓ 6 sweet onions
- ✓ 1/4 cup balsamic vinegar
- ✓ 1/4 cup honey
- ✓ 1/8 teaspoon fresh chopped tarragon

Directions: Set the oven to 175°C or 350°F to preheat.
Peel onions and form 2 cross slices on the surface of the onion. Put in a casserole dish or clay cooker. Combine tarragon, honey and balsamic vinegar together. Drizzle over onions and marinate about an hour.
Bake until onions are softened, or for about 30-40 minutes.

GRILLED FISH

Serv.: 4| **Prep.:** 10m | **Cook:** 10m

Ingredients:
- ✓ 1/4 cup olive oil
- ✓ 1 tablespoon dried parsley
- ✓ 2 tablespoons dried thyme
- ✓ 1 tablespoon dried rosemary
- ✓ 1 clove garlic, minced
- ✓ 4 (6 ounce) fillets salmon
- ✓ 1 lemon, juiced

Directions: Prepare the grill by preheating to medium heat.
Combine the garlic, rosemary, thyme, parsley, and olive oil in a shallow glass dish. Add the salmon in the dish, flipping to coat. Squeeze lemon juice over each fillet. Cover and refrigerate for 30 minutes to marinate.
Put oil lightly on the grill grate. Place salmon on the grill and get rid of any left marinade. Cook salmon on the preheated grill for 8-10 minutes over medium heat, flipping once. Fish is cooked once it flakes easily using a fork.

LAMB WITH SHIRAZ HONEY SAUCE

Serv.: 4| **Prep.:** 20m | **Cook:** 30m

Ingredients:
- ✓ 1 (7 bone) rack of lamb, trimmed and frenched
- ✓ Sea salt to taste
- ✓ 2 1/2 tablespoons ras el hanout
- ✓ 1 cup Shiraz wine
- ✓ 1/3 cup honey

Directions: Set the oven to 400°F (200°C) and start preheating.
Season lamb with sea salt; rub ras el hanout over it. Sear lamb on all sides in a medium cast iron skillet over medium-high heat until evenly browned.
Put the skillet with lamb in the prepared oven; roast for half an hour or until the internal temperature reached 145°F (63°C) as the minimum.
Take the lamb out of the skillet; reserve the juices; let stand for 10-15 minutes before you slice the ribs. Put the skillet with juices over medium heat; stir in honey and wine. Cook until the liquid reduces by about 1/2. Drizzle over ribs; serve.

SPICY CARROT SALAD

Serv.: 6| **Prep.:** 15m | **Cook:** 20m

Ingredients:

- ✓ 1 pound carrots, peeled and sliced into thin rounds
- ✓ 2 cups water
- ✓ 2 cloves garlic, minced
- ✓ 2 tablespoons olive oil
- ✓ 1/2 teaspoon sweet paprika
- ✓ 1 pinch cayenne pepper, or to taste
- ✓ Salt and ground black pepper to taste
- ✓ 1 tablespoon wine vinegar
- ✓ 1/2 teaspoon ground cumin
- ✓ 1/4 cup cilantro leaves

Directions: On medium-high heat, boil water, black pepper, carrots, salt, garlic, cayenne pepper, paprika, and olive oil together in a shallow pan for 20m until the water evaporates and the carrots are tender.

Mix cumin and vinegar into the carrot mixture. Take off pan from heat then let set aside and let the mixture cool to room temperature.

Add cilantro on top then serve.

Murphy Steaks

Serv.: 4| **Prep.:** 30m | **Cook:** 10m

Ingredients:
- ✓ 2 pounds beef tenderloin steaks
- ✓ 1 bulb garlic, cloves separated and peeled
- ✓ Salt to taste
- ✓ Ground black pepper to taste

Directions: Remove garlic clove from the bulb and peel, then cut into strips lengthwise.

Punch holes into steak using a sharp knife, then stuff garlic strips into holes. Cover and put it in the refrigerator for at least 4 hours.

Preheat grill to hot heat.

Oil the grate lightly. Put the steaks stuffed with garlic on hot grill with garlic stuff up. Cook for 4 to 5 minutes. Turn and use pepper and salt to season. Continue cooking for another 4 to 5 minutes until done.

Mushrooms and Spinach Italian Style

Serv.: 4| **Prep.:** 20m | **Cook:** 10m

Ingredients:
- ✓ 4 tablespoons olive oil
- ✓ 1 small onion, chopped
- ✓ 2 cloves garlic, chopped
- ✓ 14 ounces fresh mushrooms, sliced
- ✓ 10 ounces clean fresh spinach, roughly chopped
- ✓ 2 tablespoons balsamic vinegar
- ✓ 1/2 cup white wine
- ✓ Salt and freshly ground black pepper to taste
- ✓ Chopped fresh parsley, for garnish

Directions: In a big skillet, heat olive oil on moderately high heat. Sauté garlic and onion in the oil until they begin to soften.

Put in mushrooms and fry for 3-4 minutes, until they start to shrink. Toss in the spinach and fry until wilted, while stirring continuously, or for a several minutes.

Put in vinegar while stirring continuously until it is absorbed, then stir in white wine. Lower heat to low and simmer until the wine has nearly fully absorbed.

Season to taste with pepper and salt, then sprinkle over with fresh parsley. Serve hot.

Mussels in a Fennel and White Wine Broth

Serv.: 4| **Prep.:** 10m | **Cook:** 45m

Ingredients:
- ✓ 1 tablespoon olive oil
- ✓ 1 bulb fennel, trimmed and thickly sliced
- ✓ 1 1/2 tablespoons olive oil
- ✓ 3 cloves garlic, thinly sliced
- ✓ 1 pound mussels, cleaned and debearded
- ✓ 1 cup halved cherry tomatoes
- ✓ 1/2 cup white wine
- ✓ 1/4 cup chopped fresh flat-leaf parsley

Directions: Start heating oven to 400 deg F or 200 deg C. Put a silicone baking mat or parchment paper on a baking sheet to line.

Put fennel slices in a bowl. Over fennel, add 1 tablespoon olive oil and mix to coat. Put on the prepared baking sheet, then into the heated oven, roast for 25 to 35 minutes until fennel is heated through and becoming caramelize.

Over medium-high temperature, heat 1 1/2 tablespoons olive oil in a large skillet. Put in garlic and cook 1 to 2 minutes. Stir frequently until garlic becomes fragrant and turns light golden in color. Add mussels to garlic and toss to evenly mix. Pour in cherry tomatoes, roasted fennel, and white wine. Heat to a boil, put lid on, and cook for 3 to 5 minutes or until mussels open. Mix parsley in and serve.

GOULASH

Serv.: 6| **Prep.:** 25m | **Cook:** 35m

Ingredients:
- ✓ 1 pound lean ground beef
- ✓ 1 (8 ounce) package fresh mushrooms, sliced
- ✓ 1 green bell pepper, cut into 1/2 inch pieces
- ✓ 1 red bell pepper, cut into 1/2 inch pieces
- ✓ 1 zucchini, thickly sliced
- ✓ 1 small red onion, sliced
- ✓ 4 tablespoons olive oil
- ✓ 1/2 tablespoon paprika
- ✓ 1/2 tablespoon dried basil
- ✓ 1 teaspoon garlic salt
- ✓ 1/2 teaspoon white pepper
- ✓ 1 (14.5 ounce) can whole peeled tomatoes with liquid, chopped

Directions: Brown ground beef in a big frying pan. Take the beef out using a slotted spoon and remove the fat.
Put the frying pan into the stove again. Add in olive oil and heat over medium-high heat. Mix in pepper, garlic salt, basil, paprika, onion, squash, red and green peppers, and mushrooms. Cook for 5 minutes, you can stir it occasionally.

Lower the heat to medium. Mix in tomatoes and beef; simmer for 20 minutes, you stir it occasionally.

NETTLES

Serv.: 4| **Prep.:** 10m | **Cook:** 7m

Ingredients:
- ✓ 1/2 cup olive oil
- ✓ 1/3 cup water
- ✓ 5 cloves garlic, minced
- ✓ 5 cups nettle leaves, stalks trimmed off
- ✓ Salt and ground black pepper to taste

Directions: In a big skillet, heat olive oil with water on medium heat. Put in garlic, then simmer for approximately 2 minutes until aromatic. Lower the heat slightly and blend in nettle leaves with a wooden spoon. Cook for around 5 minutes while stirring frequently, until leaves are softened and emerald green in color. Season with pepper and salt.

NO TOMATO PASTA SAUCE

Serv.: 8| **Prep.:** 5m | **Cook:** 45m

Ingredients:
- ✓ 2 (15 ounce) cans sliced carrots, drained
- ✓ 1 (15 ounce) can sliced beets, drained
- ✓ 1 tablespoon olive oil
- ✓ 4 cloves garlic, minced
- ✓ 1 onion, chopped
- ✓ 1 bay leaf
- ✓ 2 tablespoons Italian seasoning
- ✓ 1/4 cup red wine vinegar

Directions: One can at a time, put beets and carrots in blender; blend till smooth. In skillet, heat olive oil on medium heat; mix and cook onions and garlic till onions are translucent. Mix pureed beets and carrots in; add red wine vinegar, Italian seasoning and bay leaf. Cover; cook till sauce starts to boil. Remove lid; lower heat to low. Simmer for at least 30 minutes or for up to 4 hours.

TOMATO FREE MARINARA SAUCE

Serv.: 2| Prep.: 25m | Cook: 32m

Ingredients:
- ✓ 1/4 kabocha squash, peeled and cut into small cubes
- ✓ 3 carrots, cut into small cubes
- ✓ 1/2 red beet, cut into small cubes
- ✓ 1 1/2 teaspoons olive oil
- ✓ 1/3 yellow onion, finely chopped
- ✓ 1 clove garlic, minced
- ✓ 5 leaves fresh sage, finely chopped
- ✓ 1 tablespoon capers (optional)
- ✓ 1 tablespoon dried Italian herbs
- ✓ 1 pinch Himalayan salt to taste
- ✓ 1/2 cup water, or more if needed
- ✓ 1/2 lemon, juiced
- ✓ 5 leaves fresh basil, chopped

Directions: In food processor, mix beet, carrots and kabocha squash; pulse till roughly grated.
In a saucepan, heat olive oil till sizzling over medium heat. Put in sage, garlic and onion; cook and mix for a minute, or till onion is aromatic. Mix in salt, Italian herbs, capers and grated kabocha squash mixture.
In the saucepan, put the water. Place cover on and let sauce simmer for half an hour, putting additional water if necessary, or till kabocha squash mixture is tender. Using a fork, crush mixture to create a smoother sauce.
Mix basil and lemon juice into sauce and allow the flavors to blend for a minute.

NORI CHIPS

Serv.: 2| Prep.: 5m | Cook: 5m

Ingredients:
- ✓ 1 sheet nori (dried seaweed), cut into thin strips
- ✓ 1 teaspoon olive oil, or as needed
- ✓ Salt to taste

Directions: Start preheating oven to 150 degrees C (300 degrees F). Spray baking sheet lightly with oil.

On the prepared baking sheet, place nori smooth-side down. Lightly brush nori with olive oil; add salt.
In the preheated oven, bake for 3 to 4 minutes until nori is dry and crispy.

AVOCADO & PISTACHIOS

Serv.: 2| Prep.: 10m | Cook: 0

Ingredients:
- ✓ 1 tablespoon shelled pistachios
- ✓ 1 tablespoon almonds
- ✓ 3/4 cup unsweetened coconut milk
- ✓ 5 cubes ice cubes
- ✓ 1/2 large avocado, peeled and pitted
- ✓ 1 tablespoon honey
- ✓ 1 pinch saffron threads (optional)

Directions: In a blender, blend almonds and pistachios until ground; put in saffron, honey avocado, ice cubes, and coconut milk. Blend until smooth.

PALEO KALE CHIPS

Serv.: 4| Prep.: 5m | Cook: 20m

Ingredients:
- ✓ Olive oil cooking spray
- ✓ 1 bunch kale, ribs removed and leaves torn into pieces
- ✓ 1 tablespoon coconut oil
- ✓ 1 pinch garlic salt, or to taste
- ✓ Salt and ground black pepper to taste

Directions: Heat oven to 230 degrees Celsius or 450 degrees Fahrenheit. Use cooking spray to grease a baking sheet.
Place kale and coconut oil in a bowl. Toss using your hands until coated. Place the kale on the baking sheet. Sprinkle pepper, salt, and garlic salt on top of the kale.
Put baking sheet in the oven and turn it off. Place the kale for 20 minutes in the oven until crisp.

PALEO MAPLE BACON MINI DONUTS

Serv.: 13| Prep.: 20m | Cook: 14m

Ingredients:
- ✓ 3 slices bacon, or more to taste
- ✓ 1 cup cassava flour (such as Otto's)
- ✓ 1 teaspoon baking powder
- ✓ 1/4 teaspoon salt
- ✓ 1/4 cup butter, at room temperature
- ✓ 2 tablespoons coconut sugar
- ✓ 3/4 cup coconut milk, at room temperature
- ✓ 1/4 cup maple syrup, at room temperature
- ✓ 1 egg, at room temperature
- ✓ 1/2 teaspoon vanilla extract
- ✓ Topping:
- ✓ 6 tablespoons almond butter, at room temperature
- ✓ 3 tablespoons maple syrup, at room temperature
- ✓ 2 tablespoons coconut milk, at room temperature (optional)

Directions: Put bacon in a big skillet and cook on medium-high heat for 10 minutes and turn occasionally or until it's evenly browned. Use paper towels to drain bacon slices. Reserve the bacon drippings in the skillet. Chop the bacon.
Mix salt, baking powder, and cassava flour in a bowl.
Mix coconut sugar and butter with an electric mixer in a bowl until fluffy. Add egg, 1/4 cup of maple syrup, and 3/4 cup of coconut milk mix until fully combined. Mix the flour mix in butter mix until you get a smooth batter. Place in 1 tablespoon of bacon drippings at a time if the batter is very thick. Place chopped bacon in the batter.
Heat the donut maker following the manufacturer's instructions.
Move batter into a clear plastic bag and cut off a corner. Fill the donut maker with the batter following the instructions of the manufacturer. Cook it for 4-5 minutes. Place the donuts on a wire rack. Let cool for 15 minutes.
Mix 2 tablespoons of coconut milk, 3 tablespoons of maple syrup, and almond butter in a bowl until it's extremely smooth. Dip the cooled donuts in the almond butter topping.

PALEO PEACH CRISP WITH COCONUT AND SLIVERED ALMONDS

Serv.: 4| Prep.: 10m | Cook: 30

Ingredients:
- ✓ 1 (16 ounce) package frozen peach slices
- ✓ 2 tablespoons coconut sugar, divided
- ✓ 1 1/2 cups almond flour
- ✓ 1/2 cup coconut flakes
- ✓ 1 teaspoon baking powder
- ✓ 1/2 teaspoon sea salt
- ✓ 3 tablespoons unsalted butter, cubed
- ✓ 1 teaspoon vanilla extract
- ✓ 1/4 cup slivered almonds
- ✓ 1 tablespoon coconut oil, melted

Directions: Preheat an oven to 175 °C or 350 °F. In baking dish, put slices of peach.
In preheating oven, defrost the peaches for 5 minutes. Separate and scatter equally in baking dish. Scatter a tablespoon of sugar over.
In food processor, mix salt, baking powder, coconut flakes, almond flour and leftover 1 tablespoon of coconut sugar; pulse approximately five times till blended. Put the vanilla extract and butter; pulse several more times till crumbly. Put on top of peaches.
On top of flour mixture, spread slivered almonds. Drizzle top with coconut oil.
In prepped oven, bake for 22 to 25 minutes till golden brown.

PALEO PECAN MAPLE SALMON

Serv.: 4| Prep.: 15m | Cook: 15m

Ingredients:
- ✓ 4 (4 ounce) fillets salmon
- ✓ Salt and ground black pepper to taste
- ✓ 1/2 cup pecans
- ✓ 3 tablespoons pure maple syrup
- ✓ 1 tablespoon apple cider vinegar

- ✓ 1 teaspoon smoked paprika
- ✓ 1/2 teaspoon chipotle pepper powder
- ✓ 1/2 teaspoon onion powder

Directions: On a baking sheet, put salmon fillets. Use black pepper and salt to season.

In a food processor, mix together onion powder, chipotle powder, paprika, vinegar, maple syrup, and pecans, pulse until the mixture is powdery. Put the pecan mixture on top of each salmon fillet, fully cover the entire surface. Chill the covered salmon for 2-3 hours do not put a cover on.

Start preheating the oven to 425°F (220°c).

Put the salmon in the preheated oven and bake for 12-14 minutes until a fork can easily flake the fish.

PALEO SAUSAGE MEATBALLS

Serv.: 4| **Prep.:** 25m | **Cook:** 6m

Ingredients:
- ✓ 1 apple, chopped
- ✓ 1 onion, chopped
- ✓ 2 tablespoons chopped fresh sage
- ✓ 2 tablespoons chopped fresh rosemary
- ✓ 1/2 teaspoon sea salt
- ✓ 1 pound ground sausage
- ✓ 2 tablespoons olive oil

Directions: In a food processor, mix together the sea salt, rosemary, sage, onion and apple, then pulse until combined well. Add sausage and pulse for 3-4 times until blended.

Roll the sausage mixture into meatballs.

In a big skillet, heat the olive oil on medium heat. Cook the meatballs by batches for 3-4 minutes on each side, with a cover, until it turns brown.

PALEO SEAFOOD CHILI

Serv.: 6| **Prep.:** 20m | **Cook:** 30m

Ingredients:
- ✓ 1 tablespoon olive oil
- ✓ 1 large onion, chopped
- ✓ 1 red bell pepper, chopped
- ✓ 1 green bell pepper, chopped
- ✓ 2 stalks celery, chopped
- ✓ 3 cloves garlic, minced
- ✓ 1 1/2 teaspoons sea salt, divided
- ✓ 1 teaspoon freshly ground pepper, divided
- ✓ 1 (15 ounce) can diced tomatoes
- ✓ 1 cup chicken broth
- ✓ 1 tablespoon dried parsley
- ✓ 2 teaspoons chili powder
- ✓ 3/4 teaspoon cayenne pepper
- ✓ 1 tablespoon tomato paste
- ✓ 1/2 pound sea scallops - rinsed, drained, patted dry, and cut in half
- ✓ 1/2 pound haddock, cut into cubes
- ✓ 1/2 pound uncooked medium shrimp, peeled and deveined

Directions: Heat olive oil at medium-high heat in a large heavy saucepan. Put in garlic, celery, green bell pepper, red bell pepper, and onion; cook until soft, 3 to 4 minutes. Flavor with 1/2 teaspoon of pepper and 1/2 teaspoon of salt. Put in tomatoes and broth; heat to a boil. Lower the heat to medium-low. Put in cayenne pepper, chili powder, and parsley; cook until thickened, for 15 minutes. Blend in tomato paste until dissolved.

Add the remaining 1 teaspoon of salt and 1/2 teaspoon of pepper to flavor the scallop and haddock; add to the saucepan. Mix in shrimp; cook until it is opaque in the center and bright pink on the outside, about 7 minutes.

BOOK 3

PALEO DIET FOR KIDS

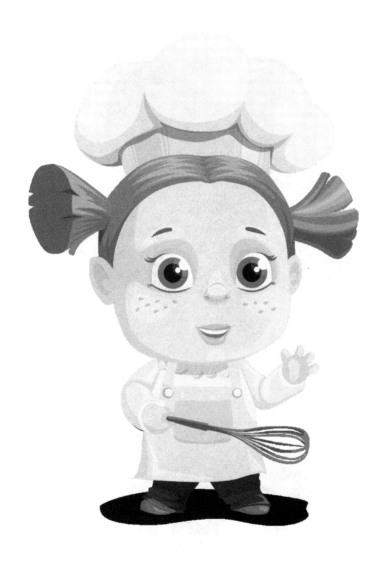

CAPRESE STUFFED ZUCCHINI

Serv.: 6| **Prep.:** 20m | **Cook:** 40m

Ingredients:
- ✓ 2 large zucchinis, halved lengthwise and seeded
- ✓ Sea salt to taste
- ✓ Freshly ground black pepper to taste
- ✓ Extra-virgin olive oil, or to taste
- ✓ 2 (1/2 inch thick) slices eggplant
- ✓ 1 cup cherry tomatoes, quartered
- ✓ 1 clove garlic, minced
- ✓ 1 cup fresh basil leaves, divided
- ✓ 1 teaspoon sea salt
- ✓ 1/2 teaspoon ground black pepper
- ✓ 3 tablespoons extra-virgin olive oil, plus more for drizzling
- ✓ 1 tablespoon balsamic vinegar

Directions: Turn the oven to 350°F (175°C) to preheat. Line a parchment paper into a baking sheet.
Use freshly ground black pepper and sea salt to season zucchini. Drizzle over the zucchini halves with 2 tablespoons of olive oil.
In the preheated oven, bake the zucchini for 10 minutes until tender. Transfer to a plate to cool; slice into 2-in. segments, keep them to stay together to look like whole halves.
Use pepper and salt to season both sides of eggplant slices, put on the baking sheet.
Bake the eggplant for 15 minutes, turn over, and keep baking for another 15-20 minutes until turning brown; transfer to a cutting board and cool briefly.
Peel and dispose the skin of the eggplant. Cut eggplant flesh and remove to a big mixing bowl; add garlic and tomatoes.
Cut 3/4 cup basil leaves; put on the eggplant mixture and use 1/2 teaspoon black pepper and 1 teaspoon salt to season. Drizzle over the mixture with 3 tablespoons olive oil; mix to blend. On the zucchini halves, put the mixture. Drizzle over the stuffed zucchini with extra olive oil and balsamic vinegar. Shred the leftover basil leaves and sprinkle them over the zucchinis.

CARAMELIZED FENNEL

Serv.: 6| **Prep.:** 10m | **Cook:** 45m

Ingredients:
- ✓ 2 bulbs fennel
- ✓ 2 tablespoons coconut oil
- ✓ 1/2 teaspoon sea salt, or to taste
- ✓ 1/3 cup white wine, divided
- ✓ 1/4 cup water, or as needed
- ✓ 1 tablespoon balsamic vinegar, or more to taste

Directions: Cut off white bulbs from the bottom of each fennel bulb. If desired, you can reserve the green tops for other purposes. Quarter each of the fennel bulbs and remove their core. Slice each bulb thinly across their grain.
In a cast-iron skillet, melt the coconut oil over high heat. Sauté the fennel for 3-5 minutes until browned lightly. Season the fennel with salt.
Add 1-2 tbsp. of wine into the skillet. Bring the mixture to a boil, from the bottom of the pan, using a wooden spoon to scrape off any browned bits of food. Adjust the heat to low. Simmer the mixture for about 40 minutes, pouring in more wine and water if necessary until the fennel is tender and golden brown.
Take the skillet away from the heat. Toss in balsamic vinegar with the fennel.

CARAMELIZED ONIONS

Serv.: 4| **Prep.:** 10m | **Cook:** 25m

Ingredients:
- ✓ 6 slices bacon, chopped
- ✓ 2 sweet onions, cut into thin strips
- ✓ 2 tablespoons molasses
- ✓ 1/4 teaspoon salt
- ✓ 1/4 teaspoon pepper

Directions: In a heavy skillet, add bacon and cook on moderately high heat until crisp. Take out the bacon and save 1 tbsp. drippings in the skillet. Crumble bacon and set aside.

In the reserved drippings, cook onions until tender and caramel colored, or for about 15 minutes. Stir in pepper, salt and molasses. Put in a serving dish and sprinkle over with crumbled bacon.

CARIBBEAN COCONUT CHICKEN

Serv.: 4| **Prep.:** 20m | **Cook:** 1h

Ingredients:
- ✓ 4 skinless, boneless chicken breasts
- ✓ 1 teaspoon vegetable oil
- ✓ 1 1/2 onions, chopped
- ✓ 1 red bell pepper, chopped
- ✓ 1 green bell pepper, chopped
- ✓ 1 tablespoon chopped roasted garlic
- ✓ 1/2 (14 ounce) can coconut milk
- ✓ Salt and pepper to taste
- ✓ 1 pinch crushed red pepper flakes

Directions: Prepare the oven by preheating to 425°F (220°C).
Fry chicken breast in vegetable oil in a big skillet until the chicken just starts to brown.
Mix red and green bell peppers, and onions in the skillet with chicken. Stir-fry until the onions are glassy. Once the vegetables become translucent, mix in the coconut milk and garlic. Cook mixture for 5-8 minutes then take off heat. Add red pepper flakes, pepper, and salt to season.
Place the mixture in a 9x13-inch baking dish and place in the preheated oven then bake for 45 minutes at 425°F (220°C), or until the chicken becomes tender and vegetables cook down.

CARIBBEAN HEALTH DRINK

Serv.: 2| **Prep.:** 10m | **Cook:** 0

Ingredients:
- ✓ 1 cup chopped carrot
- ✓ 1 banana
- ✓ 1 kiwi, peeled
- ✓ 1 apple - peeled, cored, and sliced
- ✓ 1 cup chopped pineapple
- ✓ 1 cup ice cubes

Directions: Throw ice cubes and pieces of banana, kiwi, pineapple, apple, and carrot in a food processor or blender and process until smooth.

CHICKEN KABOBS MEXICANA

Serv.: 4| **Prep.:** 30m | **Cook:** 10m

Ingredients:
- ✓ 2 tablespoons olive oil
- ✓ 1 teaspoon ground cumin
- ✓ 2 tablespoons chopped fresh cilantro
- ✓ 1 lime, juiced
- ✓ Salt and ground black pepper to taste
- ✓ 2 skinless, boneless chicken breast halves - cut into 1 inch cubes
- ✓ 1 small zucchini, cut into 1/2-inch slices
- ✓ 1 onion, cut into wedges and separated
- ✓ 1 red bell pepper, cut into 1 inch pieces
- ✓ 10 cherry tomatoes

Directions: Combine olive oil, lime juice, cilantro, cumin, salt and pepper in a shallow dish. Put in the chicken and mix well to coat. Cover and marinate in the refrigerator for one hour, minimum.
Preheat grill on high.
Cue the chicken, tomatoes, zucchini, bell peppers, and onions onto skewers.
Lightly oil the grates. Grill the skewers, turning to cook chicken evenly for 10 minutes or until cooked through.

CHICKEN STOCK

Serv.: 14| **Prep.:** 20m| **Cook:** 4h

Ingredients:
- ✓ 4 pounds chicken
- ✓ 7 cups water
- ✓ 1 large onion, halved
- ✓ 3 stalks celery
- ✓ 3 carrots, cut into 2 inch pieces
- ✓ 1 bay leaf
- ✓ 1 teaspoon grated fresh ginger
- ✓ Salt to taste

Directions: Add the chicken to a big pot over high heat. Pour in water to cover and boil them up; lower to medium-low heat and let simmer for 60 minutes.

Take the chicken out from the pot, leave water there. Let chicken cool. Take out bones and skin out from the meat. Take the skins and bones back to the pot. Add salt, ginger, bay leaf, celery, carrots and onions. Keep simmering for 3 to 4 hours. Filter the stock through a strainer and let cool, uncovered.

The chicken meat can be used for sandwiches, salads, soups or whatever needs chicken. Remove any fat from the stock then use or store in freezer right away. Store it in one-cup amounts and replace water while making gravy, vegetables or rice.

CITRUS SHRIMP

Serv.: 6 | **Prep.:** 45m | **Cook:** 5m

Ingredients:
- ✓ 2 oranges, zested and juiced
- ✓ 3 limes, zested and juiced
- ✓ 2 tablespoons olive oil
- ✓ 1/2 teaspoon salt, or to taste
- ✓ 3 cloves garlic
- ✓ 1 1/2 pounds large shrimp, peeled and deveined

Directions: Mix together salt, garlic, olive oil, lime zest and juice, orange zest and juice in a food processor or blender. Be careful as the shrimp can suck salt. Puree with cover until it is smoothened. In a bowl, add shrimp and citrus marinade. Leave them at room temperature for 20 minutes to marinate.

Over medium-high heat, heat a non-stick skillet. Add shrimp and fry each side for 3 minutes until they turn opaque. If necessary, cook in batches. While cooking, add a little of marinade to the skillet for extra flavor if desired.

CITRUS SLUSH

Serv.: 4 | **Prep.:** 5m | **Cook:** 0

Ingredients:
- ✓ 1 orange, peeled and chopped
- ✓ 1 lime, peeled and chopped
- ✓ 12 cubes ice

Directions: Mix ice cubes, lime and orange in a blender. Blend until smooth then chill for about 5 minutes. Transfer into glasses to serve.

CURRIED BUTTERNUT SQUASH SOUP

Serv.: 4 | **Prep.:** 15m | **Cook:** 1h20m

Ingredients:
- ✓ 1 butternut squash
- ✓ 1 tablespoon olive oil, or as needed
- ✓ 1 onion, chopped
- ✓ 1 shallot, minced
- ✓ 2 tablespoons curry powder, or more to taste
- ✓ 1 teaspoon ground turmeric
- ✓ 1 apple, cored and chopped
- ✓ 1 slice fresh ginger, minced
- ✓ Water to cover
- ✓ 1 (14 ounce) can coconut milk
- ✓ Salt to taste

Directions: Preheat the oven to 350°F (175°C). Put the butternut squash on a baking sheet, and pierce it.

Let it bake for 45 minutes in the preheated oven until tender. Be sure it has cooled down enough before handling. Once ready, slice it in half, remove the seeds and peel the skin. Chop the flesh.

In a skillet, heat olive oil over medium heat. Sauté onions and shallots for 10 minutes, until soft and translucent. Add and cook the turmeric and curry powder for 2 minutes. Make sure everything is evenly coated.

Add apple, ginger, and squash to the onion mixture. Pour water in to cover everything. Let it boil. Then lower the heat to a medium-low. Let it simmer for about 15 minutes, until the apples and squash have become tender. Use a potato masher or immersion blender to blend the squash until it is broken up.

Pour coconut milk and add salt. Let it simmer for 3 minutes, until it is heated through.

CLAMATO® SHRIMP "CEVICHE" STYLE

Serv.: 4| **Prep.:** 15m | **Cook:** 0

Ingredients:
- ✓ 2 pounds cooked shrimp
- ✓ 1 small red onion, thinly sliced
- ✓ 1 fresh jalapeno chile, seeded and minced
- ✓ 1 cucumber, peeled, seeded, thinly sliced
- ✓ 1/2 bunch cilantro, finely chopped
- ✓ 2 limes, juiced
- ✓ 1/2 cup Clamato® Tomato Cocktail

Directions: Mix cilantro, cucumber, jalapeno, onion and shrimp together in a bowl.
Add Clamato(R) and lime juice; stir well to mix.
Chill in the fridge for 20 to 30 minutes.
Serve cold with soda crackers or tostadas (hard tortillas).

CLAMS CREOLE

Serv.: 4| **Prep.:** 20m | **Cook:** 15m

Ingredients:
- ✓ 1 tablespoon olive oil
- ✓ 1/2 cup chopped green onions, white part only
- ✓ 1/2 cup finely chopped green bell pepper
- ✓ 1/2 cup finely chopped celery
- ✓ 2 teaspoons minced garlic
- ✓ 1/4 cup white wine
- ✓ 1 (10 ounce) can diced tomatoes with green chile peppers
- ✓ 2 pounds fresh cherrystone or littleneck clams, scrubbed

Directions: Over medium heat, heat the oil in a pot that is large enough to accommodate the clams.
Add the garlic, celery, green pepper and onions.
Cook while stirring for about 5 minutes until tender.
Mix in can of tomatoes along with clams, wine and green chilies. Raise the heat to medium-high, cover pot and then cook for about 5 to 8 minutes or until

all of clams are opened. Transfer from the heat right away.

CLAMS KOKKINISTO

Serv.: 6| **Prep.:** 15m | **Cook:** 1h

Ingredients:
- ✓ 1/2 cup chopped onion
- ✓ 2 large stalks celery, chopped
- ✓ 4 cloves garlic, minced
- ✓ 2 tablespoons olive oil
- ✓ 1 (28 ounce) can canned peeled and diced tomatoes
- ✓ 1 (6 ounce) can tomato paste
- ✓ 2 (7 ounce) cans whole baby clams, undrained
- ✓ 4 bay leaves
- ✓ 1/2 teaspoon chili pepper flakes
- ✓ 2 teaspoons dried oregano
- ✓ Salt and pepper to taste
- ✓ 2 tablespoons olive oil

Directions: Sauté garlic, celery and onion in 2 tablespoons of the olive oil in large saucepan, until tender. Mix in clams, tomato paste and tomatoes. Season to taste with pepper, salt, oregano, chili pepper flakes and bay leaves. Simmer, covered, until sauce thickens and tomatoes' color start to turn deep red, about 60 m. Stir in the remaining two tablespoons of the olive oil near the end of cooking time.

CRANBERRY SALAD

Serv.: 7| **Prep.:** 10m | **Cook:** 0

Ingredients:
- ✓ 2 cups cranberries
- ✓ 1 large orange
- ✓ 1 cup white sugar
- ✓ 1 cup finely chopped walnuts
- ✓ 1 cup chopped celery
- ✓ 1 cup crushed pineapple, drained
- ✓ 1 (3 ounce) package raspberry flavored Jell-O® mix
- ✓ 2 cups hot water

Directions: Mix hot water with the gelatin (do not

let stand). Crush the orange and cranberries, rind included, and mix it with sugar. Incorporate pineapple, celery and nuts. Combine with the prepared gelatin mixture and chill.

CRANBERRY THOKKU

Serv.: 8| **Prep.:** 5m | **Cook:** 6m

Ingredients:
- ✓ 2 tablespoons olive oil
- ✓ 1 teaspoon mustard seeds
- ✓ 1 teaspoon fenugreek seeds
- ✓ 1/8 teaspoon ground turmeric
- ✓ 1/8 teaspoon asafoetida powder
- ✓ 1 (12 ounce) package fresh cranberries, finely chopped
- ✓ 1 teaspoon salt
- ✓ 1/2 teaspoon achar masala

Directions: In a saucepan, heat asafoetida, turmeric, fenugreek seeds, mustard seeds, and olive oil over medium heat; stir for about 1 minute until aromatic. Stir in achar masala, salt, and cranberries; cook, stirring, for 5 to 7 minutes until cranberries are tender and break down. Take away from heat and allow to cool before serving.

DUCK ROASTED BRUSSELS SPROUTS

Serv.: 4| **Prep.:** 20m | **Cook:** 15m

Ingredients:
- ✓ 2 tablespoons duck fat, or more as needed
- ✓ 2 pounds Brussels sprouts, trimmed and halved lengthwise
- ✓ Salt and freshly ground black pepper to taste
- ✓ 1 pinch cayenne pepper, or more to taste
- ✓ 1 lemon, juiced

Directions: Preheat the oven to 450°F (230°C). Use silicone baking mat or parchment paper to line the baking sheet. In a small saucepan, insert the duck fat and heat until it melts. Mix the melted duck fat, cayenne pepper, black pepper, salt and Brussels sprouts together in a big bowl, tossing to coat the Brussels sprouts evenly. Move the sprouts into the prepped baking sheet and put it into the preheated oven. Leave them baking for 15 to 20 minutes until the Brussels sprouts tenderize and brown while maintaining some firmness. Midway through the process, turn the sprouts around. Finish off by adding fresh lemon juice that has just been squeezed over the top.

DYNAMITES

Serv.: 6| **Prep.:** 15m | **Cook:** 4-6h

Ingredients:
- ✓ 2 teaspoons vegetable oil
- ✓ 1 onion, chopped
- ✓ 2 pounds ground beef
- ✓ 4 green bell peppers, chopped
- ✓ 1 (14.5 ounce) can diced tomatoes
- ✓ 1 (8 ounce) can tomato sauce
- ✓ 1 (6 ounce) can tomato paste
- ✓ 1 teaspoon crushed red pepper flakes (optional)

Directions: In a saucepan, heat oil over medium-high heat. In hot oil, cook onion for 5 m or until tender. Put red pepper flakes, tomato paste, tomato sauce, tomatoes, bell peppers and ground beef into saucepan, then stir.
Lower the heat to medium-low and simmer for 4-6 hours until beef becomes tender and peppers become soft.

EASY MEAT SAUCE

Serv.: 6| **Prep.:** 10m | **Cook:** 1h30m

Ingredients:
- ✓ 1 tablespoon olive oil
- ✓ 1 onion, chopped
- ✓ 1 1/4 pounds ground beef
- ✓ 2 tablespoons Italian seasoning
- ✓ 2 (15 ounce) cans tomato sauce
- ✓ 2 (15 ounce) cans fire-roasted diced tomatoes
- ✓ 1 teaspoon salt
- ✓ 1 splash red wine

Directions: In a big skillet, heat olive oil on medium-high heat. Sauté onion in hot oil for about

5 minutes until it becomes soft. Use Italian seasoning to season the onion. Keep on sautéing for about 3 minutes until the herbs are fragrant. Break the beef into small pieces then put it into the skillet. Cook and stir for 5 to 7 minutes until it becomes crumbly and brown.

Mix diced tomatoes and tomato sauce into the beef mixture then use salt to season. Put the lid on the skillet then turn the heat down to low. Cook at a simmer 1 hour.

Splash the wine on top of the mixture, mix, and simmer for about 20 minutes until it becomes thick.

Easy Pizza Sauce

Serv.: 8 | **Prep.:** 10m | **Cook:** 0

Ingredients:
- ✓ 1 (6 ounce) can tomato paste
- ✓ 1 1/2 cups water
- ✓ 1/3 cup extra virgin olive oil
- ✓ 2 cloves garlic, minced
- ✓ Salt to taste
- ✓ Ground black pepper to taste
- ✓ 1/2 tablespoon dried oregano
- ✓ 1/2 tablespoon dried basil
- ✓ 1/2 teaspoon dried rosemary, crushed

Directions: Combine olive oil, water and tomato paste together then mix well. Put in rosemary, basil, oregano, garlic, salt and pepper to taste. Blend well and allow to stand for a few hours to allow flavors to combine. Just spread on dough, no need to cook.

Easy Roasted Cabbage

Serv.: 6 | **Prep.:** 10m | **Cook:** 40m

Ingredients:
- ✓ 1 head cabbage, sliced into six 1-inch pieces
- ✓ 6 tablespoons olive oil
- ✓ Salt and ground black pepper to taste

Directions: Set the oven to 220°C or 425°F to preheat.

Use olive oil to brush both sides of each cabbage piece and season with black pepper and salt. Place on a baking sheet in a single layer.

In the preheated oven, bake about 40-55 minutes, until softened.

Easy Salmon

Serv.: 4 | **Prep.:** 10m | **Cook:** 6m

Ingredients:
- ✓ 1 pound salmon fillets, skin removed
- ✓ 1/2 white onion, thinly sliced
- ✓ 1/2 tomato, diced
- ✓ 1 tablespoon garlic powder, or to taste
- ✓ 1 tablespoon onion powder, or to taste
- ✓ 2 tablespoons white wine
- ✓ 2 tablespoons extra-virgin olive oil
- ✓ Sea salt and fresh black pepper to taste

Directions: Transfer salmon fillets to a microwave-safe baking dish of 8x8-inch, and then add the tomato and onion on top of the fillets. Drizzle with onion powder and garlic powder. Sprinkle olive oil and white wine on top and the use plastic wrap to wrap the dish.

Heat in microwave for about 6 minutes on High power setting until the fish becomes opaque. Remove the plastic wrap carefully to evade steam and then season to taste with pepper and salt.

Easy Slow Cooker Apple Pork Roast

Serv.: 14 | **Prep.** 15m | **Cook:** 8h

Ingredients:
- ✓ 6 apples with peel, cored and cut into 8 wedges
- ✓ 1 large red onion, roughly chopped
- ✓ 1/4 teaspoon ground cinnamon, or to taste
- ✓ 7 pounds pork shoulder roast
- ✓ 1/2 teaspoon salt, or to taste
- ✓ 1/2 teaspoon ground black pepper, or to taste
- ✓ 1 (24 ounce) jar cinnamon-flavored applesauce
- ✓ 1/4 teaspoon ground cinnamon, or to taste

Directions: Arrange onion and apples to the

bottom of a slow cooker, and add on top a quarter teaspoon of cinnamon.

Rub pepper and salt all over the pork roast, then lay on top of onion-apple layer in the slow cooker. Pour applesauce onto the roast and top with a quarter teaspoon of cinnamon.

Cook for 8 hours over high setting. Place onions, apples and sauce onto the roast and serve.

EASY SMOKED TURKEY

Serv.: 12| **Prep.:** 20m | **Cook:** 4h

Ingredients:
- ✓ 1 (12 pound) thawed whole turkey, neck and giblets removed
- ✓ 1 tablespoon chopped fresh savory
- ✓ 1 tablespoon chopped fresh sage
- ✓ 1 tablespoon salt (optional)
- ✓ 1 tablespoon ground black pepper
- ✓ 1/8 cup olive oil
- ✓ 1/2 cup water

Directions: Wash turkey and using paper towels, pat it dry. In a bowl, mix black pepper, salt, sage and savory; massage 1/2 of herb mix on the inside of turkey's cavity and neck cavity. Loosen turkey skin on legs and breast; massage the leftover 1/2 of herb mixture beneath the loosened skin. Massage the olive oil all over the turkey.

Light 20 charcoal briquettes and on lower grate of kettle charcoal grill, put 1/2 of them on every side. Put a disposable aluminum baking pan or drip pan in the center of lower grate and add water. Once coals turn gray with ash, put a 2-inch square piece of hickory or different hardwood onto every coals' bank.

Over cooking grate, put the turkey and place cover on grill. Using grill thermometer, check the temperature to keep heat between 65 to 120°C or 150 and 250°F; put in about 3 to 5 coals to every side approximately every 1 1/2 hours. Once hardwood pieces burn away, put in additional to maintain a consistent stream of smoke rising from wood. In case open flames erupt once you open the lid, extinguish them with a drizzle of beer or water.

Let the turkey smoke for approximately 4 hours total, 20 minutes each pound; allow the temperature to raise to 120°C or 250°F on the final hour of smoking. An inserted instant-read meat thermometer into the chunkiest part of a thigh without touching bone should register 75°C or 165°F.

EASY VEGAN PASTA SAUCE

Serv.: 3| **Prep.:** 15m | **Cook:** 20m

Ingredients:
- ✓ 1 teaspoon vegetable oil
- ✓ 1/2 small yellow onion, diced
- ✓ 2 cloves garlic, minced
- ✓ 5 large tomatoes, cubed
- ✓ 1 small green bell pepper, diced
- ✓ 1/2 teaspoon salt
- ✓ 1/2 teaspoon black pepper
- ✓ 1 teaspoon dried basil leaves
- ✓ 1/2 teaspoon dried oregano

Directions: In a skillet, sauté garlic and onion with vegetable oil over medium-low heat. Place in the tomatoes and stir in oregano, basil, pepper, salt, and diced bell pepper. Allow to simmer, stirring sometimes, for 20 minutes. If it starts to stick, bring the heat down.

EGGPLANT AND TOMATO PACKETS

Serv.: 2| **Prep.:** 5m | **Cook:** 20m

Ingredients:
- ✓ 1 eggplant, peeled and halved lengthwise
- ✓ 1 tomato, halved
- ✓ 1 pinch garlic salt
- ✓ Ground black pepper to taste
- ✓ 2 teaspoons olive oil
- ✓ 2 sheets heavy duty aluminum foil

Directions: Preheat outdoor grill to medium heat. On each aluminum foil sheet, put 1 tomato half and 1 eggplant half. Sprinkle black pepper and garlic salt. Drizzle olive oil. Fold foil up to make packets.

Grill packets for 15 minutes or till tomato and eggplant are very tender.

EGGY GUACAMOLE

Serv.: 1| **Prep.:** 5m | **Cook:** 18m

Ingredients:
- ✓ 1 large egg
- ✓ 1 avocado

Directions: Put the egg in a small pot and add cold water to cover. The water should be about 1 inch or so higher than the egg. Then cover with a lid. Make your eggs to a rolling boil over high heat. Separate from heat and allow to stand for 18 minutes for medium sized eggs, 20 minutes for large eggs and 23 minutes for extra large eggs. Then drain water and instantly run cold water over eggs until cooled.
Quick cooling helps prevent a green ring from forming around the yolks. Peel eggs and put in a bowl. Crush well and reserve.
Slice avocado in half, take off the pit and spoon out flesh. Put avocado flesh in a bowl and use fork to mash well. Mix avocado and egg together and mash well until you reach the desired consistency.

FRESH HERBED HALIBUT

Serv.: 4| **Prep.:** 10m | **Cook:** 20m

Ingredients:
- ✓ 1 (2 pound) halibut fillet
- ✓ 1 large lemon, quartered
- ✓ Olive oil for brushing
- ✓ 1 teaspoon sea salt
- ✓ 1 teaspoon garlic powder
- ✓ 1 tablespoon dill weed

Directions: Preheat an oven broiler. Coat olive oil on a broiling pan/baking sheet.
Rinse fish; pat dry. Put onto greased pan. Coat olive oil cooking spray/brush olive oil on. Squeeze lemon wedges juice on entire fillet. Generously season with salt followed by garlic then dill.

In preheated oven, broil till fish can be flaked using a fork and is opaque for 15-20 minutes. The broiling time varies on the fillet's thickness.

FRESH PINEAPPLE BERRY

Serv.: 4| **Prep.:** 15m | **Cook:** 0

Ingredients:
- ✓ 2 fresh pineapples, peeled, cored and cubed
- ✓ 4 cups fresh strawberries, washed
- ✓ 2 cups blueberries
- ✓ 1 cup ice cubes

Directions: In a juice machine, juice together blueberries, strawberries and pineapple, then pour the juice into a blender together with ice cubes. Puree until smooth.

FRESH ROSEMARY LANGOSTINO SALAD

Serv.: 4| **Prep.:** 15m | **Cook:**

Ingredients:
- ✓ 1 (16 ounce) package frozen pre-cooked langostinos (such as Trader Joe's®), thawed
- ✓ 1 red bell pepper, diced
- ✓ 1/4 cup finely chopped fresh rosemary
- ✓ 1/2 teaspoon sea salt
- ✓ 1/2 teaspoon red pepper flakes
- ✓ 1/4 cup dry white wine
- ✓ 1/4 cup white balsamic vinegar

Directions: In a large bowl, add langostinos, red bell pepper, rosemary, sea salt, red pepper flakes, white wine, and balsamic vinegar, in this order. Mix well until langostinos are evenly coated.
Cover the bowl with plastic wrap and place in the refrigerator for at least 4 hours to overnight for the flavors to blend.

FRESH TOMATO BASIL SAUCE

Serv.: 6| **Prep.:** 20m | **Cook:** 2h

Ingredients:
- ✓ 8 pounds tomatoes, seeded and diced

- ✓ 1/4 cup chopped fresh basil
- ✓ 1 large onion, minced
- ✓ 3 cloves garlic, minced
- ✓ 1/2 cup olive oil
- ✓ Salt and pepper to taste

Directions: Cook basil and tomatoes in a big saucepan over medium-low heat until tomatoes are soft.

Meanwhile, sauté garlic and onion in olive oil in a medium skillet until the onions become translucent.

Put the onion mixture into the tomato mixture. Put in pepper and salt then allow to simmer on low heat until thick or for 2 hours.

FRESH TOMATO MARINARA SAUCE

Serv.: 6| **Prep.:** 15m | **Cook:** 1h10m

Ingredients:
- ✓ 3 tablespoons olive oil
- ✓ 1/2 onion, chopped
- ✓ 8 large tomatoes, peeled and cut into big chunks
- ✓ 6 cloves garlic, minced
- ✓ 1 bay leaf
- ✓ 1/2 cup red wine
- ✓ 1 tablespoon honey
- ✓ 2 teaspoons dried basil
- ✓ 1 teaspoon oregano
- ✓ 1 teaspoon dried marjoram
- ✓ 1 teaspoon salt
- ✓ 1/2 teaspoon ground black pepper
- ✓ 1/4 teaspoon fennel seed
- ✓ 1/4 teaspoon crushed red pepper
- ✓ 2 teaspoons balsamic vinegar, or more to taste

Directions: In a stockpot over medium heat, heat olive oil. To start, cook while stirring the onion in the hot oil for 5 minutes until it becomes soft. Put in the bay leaves, garlic, and tomatoes. Boil the liquid that came from the tomatoes. Lower the heat to medium-low and leave the pot to simmer for half an hour until the tomatoes become soft. Add crushed red pepper, fennel seed, black pepper, salt, marjoram, oregano, basil, honey, and red wine to the tomato mixture and stir. Let it simmer again

for another 30 minutes to let the herbs flavor the sauce.

Finally, add balsamic vinegar to the sauce and stir well.

FRESH TURMERIC PASTE

Serv.: 12| **Prep.:** 5m | **Cook:** 10m

Ingredients:
- ✓ 2 tablespoons coconut oil
- ✓ 1 (2 inch) piece fresh turmeric root, peeled and grated
- ✓ 1 (1 inch) piece fresh ginger, peeled and grated
- ✓ 1 teaspoon fresh ground black pepper
- ✓ 1/3 cup water, divided

Directions: In a saucepan, mix together black pepper, ginger root, turmeric root, and coconut oil together; pour 1/2 of the water. Stir and cook the mixture over medium heat for 1-2 minutes until small bubbles appear around the edges. Lower the heat to medium-low; cook, tossing continuously and adding a little of the leftover water, for 5-8 minutes until the mixture turns to a paste.

Move the paste to a glass container and let cool to room temperature. Chill in the fridge with a tight cover.

FRESH AND CRISP CUCUMBER SALAD

Serv.: 4| **Prep.:** 15m | **Cook:** 0

Ingredients:
- ✓ 2 large cucumbers, peeled and sliced
- ✓ 2 large carrots, shredded
- ✓ 1 large yellow bell pepper, seeded and cut into strips
- ✓ 1 large red bell pepper, seeded and cut into strips
- ✓ 1/4 red onion, minced (optional)
- ✓ 2 teaspoons lemon zest
- ✓ 1 large lemon, juiced

Directions: In a bowl, combine red onion, red bell pepper, yellow bell pepper, carrots, and cucumbers.

Use lemon zest to sprinkle over the cucumber mixture. Drizzle over the salad with lemon juice and mix to combine. Put in a fridge until completely chilled to enjoy.

FRESH AND LIGHT CUCUMBER SALSA

Serv.: 20| **Prep.:** 25m | **Cook:**

Ingredients:
- ✓ 3 (10 ounce) cans diced tomatoes and green chilies, drained
- ✓ 3 cucumbers - peeled, seeded and chopped
- ✓ 2 roma (plum) tomatoes, chopped (or more to taste)
- ✓ 1 bunch fresh cilantro, chopped
- ✓ 1/4 cup chopped onion, or to taste
- ✓ 1 jalapeno pepper, seeded and minced, or to taste
- ✓ Kosher salt to taste

Directions: In a bowl, combine together kosher salt, jalapeno pepper, onion, cilantro, roma tomatoes, cucumbers, green chilies and diced tomatoes. Serve promptly or refrigerate for a minimum of an hour to get the best flavor.

FRICASE DE POLLO

Serv.: 3| **Prep.:** 25m | **Cook:** 15m

Ingredients:
- ✓ 1 tablespoon extra-virgin olive oil
- ✓ 1/2 large red bell pepper, diced
- ✓ 1/2 red onion, diced
- ✓ 4 cloves garlic, smashed
- ✓ 2 tablespoons tomato paste
- ✓ 2 cups water, or as needed
- ✓ 6 skinless chicken leg quarters, separated into thighs and drumsticks
- ✓ Salt to taste

Directions: In pressure cooker, heat oil on medium. Mix in onion and red bell pepper; stir and cook for 5 minutes until the onion is translucent and soft. Stir in garlic and sauté until golden.

In pressure cooker, mix a cup of water with tomato paste. Space the chicken drumsticks and thighs in the pan evenly, pour in water to cover chicken. Secure the lid and pressurize on high heat. Lower the heat to maintain full pressure, cook 15 minutes. Turn heat off and let the pressure release naturally, 20 minutes. Season with salt.

FRIED BROCCOLI

Serv.: 4| **Prep.:** 5m | **Cook:** 5m

Ingredients:
- ✓ 1 (16 ounce) package frozen broccoli, thawed
- ✓ 1 tablespoon olive oil
- ✓ 1/2 teaspoon crushed red pepper flakes
- ✓ Salt to taste

Directions: Wash and pat dry the broccoli.
In a big skillet, heat the olive oil on medium heat, then put in crushed red pepper and heat for a minute. Cook and stir in the skillet with the broccoli for 5-7 minutes, until it starts to get crispy. Season with salt and serve.

FRIED CABBAGE AND KIELBASA

Serv.: 5| **Prep.:** 10m | **Cook:** 1h15m

Ingredients:
- ✓ 6 slices bacon
- ✓ 1 head cabbage, chopped
- ✓ 1 large onion, chopped
- ✓ Salt and ground black pepper to taste
- ✓ 1 (16 oz) ring kielbasa sausage, sliced thin

Directions: In a big skillet, add bacon and cook on medium-high heat for 10 minutes while turning sometimes, until browned evenly. Transfer bacon to paper towels to drain then crumble. Save drippings in the skillet.
In the reserved bacon drippings, cook and stir onion with cabbage on medium-high heat for 1-2 minutes, until cabbage starts to wilt. Stir the cabbage mixture with pepper, salt and bacon, then cook for 3-5 minutes longer until cabbage has been wilted. Stir cabbage mixture with kielbasa and

lower heat to low. Place a cover on the skillet and simmer the cabbage mixture for an hour, until cabbage is tender and turn light golden.

FRIED CABBAGE WITH BACON

Serv.: 6| **Prep.:** 15m | **Cook:** 1h

Ingredients:
- ✓ 6 slices bacon, chopped
- ✓ 1 large onion, diced
- ✓ 2 cloves garlic, minced
- ✓ 1 large head cabbage, cored and sliced
- ✓ 1 tablespoon salt, or to taste
- ✓ 1 teaspoon ground black pepper
- ✓ 1/2 teaspoon onion powder
- ✓ 1/2 teaspoon garlic powder
- ✓ 1/8 teaspoon paprika

Directions: In a big stockpot placed on medium-high heat, cook the bacon until it becomes crisp, 10 minutes. Add the garlic and onion, stir and cook until onion is caramelized, 10 minutes. Pour in the cabbage immediately and let it cook for 10 minutes. Season with salt, garlic powder, pepper, onion powder, and paprika. Decrease to low heat, simmer while covered for half an hour, stirring often.

GARAM MASALA

Serv.: 12| **Prep.:** 5m | **Cook:** 10m

Ingredients:
- ✓ 1/3 cup cumin seeds
- ✓ 3 tablespoons coriander seeds
- ✓ 3 (4 inch) cinnamon sticks, broken into pieces
- ✓ 5 bay leaves
- ✓ 1 teaspoon nutmeg
- ✓ 5 whole star anise pods
- ✓ 14 green cardamom pods
- ✓ 1 teaspoon whole cloves
- ✓ 1 teaspoon whole black peppercorns
- ✓ 1 teaspoon ground mace

Directions: In a skillet over medium heat, toast together the mace, peppercorns, cloves, cardamom pods, anise pods, nutmeg, bay leaves, cinnamon sticks, coriander seeds and cumin seeds for 8 to 12 minutes till very aromatic and you can literally see the aroma going up into the air; take off the heat and slightly cool the mixture for approximately 10 minutes.
Into the grinder, put spice mixture; grind to make a fine powder. Keep in an airtight container.

GARAM MASALA CHICKEN

Serv.: 4| **Prep.:** 10m | **Cook:** 20m

Ingredients:
- ✓ 1 tablespoon olive oil
- ✓ 4 (3 ounce) skinless, boneless chicken breast halves
- ✓ 1 bunch green onions, chopped
- ✓ 1 1/2 cups chopped tomatoes
- ✓ 1 teaspoon garlic salt
- ✓ 1/4 cup water
- ✓ 2 teaspoons garam masala, divided

Directions: In a large skillet, heat the olive oil over medium-high heat. Put chicken breasts in the hot oil and cook for about 3 minutes, until brown on one side. Flip the chicken; put in onions and cook for 2 minutes more. Put in water, garlic salt and tomatoes, mix. Add in 1 1/2 teaspoon of garam masala to season. Heat the mixture to a boil. Lower heat to medium-low; cover and let simmer for 10 minutes, stirring occasionally.
Mix the remaining 1/2 teaspoon of garam masala through the mixture. Increase the heat to medium and heat mixture to a boil. Cook about 5 minutes more, until the juices run clear and the middle of the chicken is no longer pink. Insert an instant-read thermometer into the middle and it should read at least 165°F (74°C).

GARLIC HERB GRILLED PORK TENDERLOIN

Serv.: 4| **Prep.:** 15m | **Cook:** 1h

Ingredients:

- ✓ 3 pounds pork tenderloin
- ✓ 1/4 cup olive oil
- ✓ 3 cloves garlic, chopped
- ✓ 1/2 teaspoon chopped fresh thyme
- ✓ 1/2 tablespoon chopped fresh rosemary
- ✓ 1 tablespoon salt
- ✓ 2 tablespoons ground black pepper

Directions: Slice a slit horizontally in the pork tenderloin, making sure to leave the halves attached. Rub olive oil all over the tenderloin.
Fill the slit and the fatty side of the pork with garlic. Press the rosemary and thyme into the slit.
Sprinkle salt and pepper all over the tenderloin.
Set the outdoor grill to medium-high heat for preheating.
Put oil onto the grill grate lightly. Arrange the pork onto the grill and cook for approximately 1 hour, flipping every 15 minutes.
The minimum internal temperature of the meat must be 145°F (63°C).

GARLIC KALE

Serv.: 4| **Prep.:** 5m | **Cook:** 10m

Ingredients:
- ✓ 1 bunch kale
- ✓ 2 tablespoons olive oil
- ✓ 4 cloves garlic, minced

Directions: Tear the kale leaves into bite-size pieces from the thick stems and get rid of the stems.
In a big pot, heat olive oil on moderate heat. Cook and stir garlic in the hot oil for 2 minutes, until tender. Put in kale and keep on cooking and stirring for 5 minutes longer, until kale is wilted and bright green.

GARLIC LOVES ROASTED CABBAGE

Serv.: 8| **Prep.:** 15m | **Cook:** 40m

Ingredients:
- ✓ 1 head cabbage, or more to taste, quartered and cored

- ✓ Salt and ground black pepper to taste
- ✓ 8 cloves garlic, crushed, or to taste
- ✓ 1/4 cup olive oil, or to taste
- ✓ 1/4 cup water (optional)

Directions: Set the oven to 200°C or 400°F and set a rack in the center of the oven for preheating.
Slice each cabbage quarter into wedges with size of 1/2 inch or 1/4 inch.
Spread a big roasting pan with a half of the cabbage. Use black pepper and salt to season slightly, then scatter top with 4 cloves of garlic. Use 2 tbsp. of olive oil to drizzle over cabbage without mixing.
Place leftover cabbage in layer on top. Use black pepper and salt to season, then scatter top with the leftover garlic. Drizzle top with leftover 2 tbsp. of olive oil.
In the preheated oven, roast cabbage for 20 minutes, until it is softened a bit. Add in water in case cabbage looks dry. Keep on roasting for 20 minutes longer, until wilts.

GARLIC OIL

Serv.: 12| **Prep.:** 5m | **Cook:** 0

Ingredients:
- ✓ 8 cloves garlic
- ✓ 2 cups extra-virgin olive oil

Directions: Use back of knife to crush garlic cloves on flat surface; discard peel. Put olive oil in jar. Add garlic cloves and cover. Refrigerate for 2-5 days till flavors blend.

GARLIC PRIME RIB

Serv.: 15| **Prep.:** 10m | **Cook:** 1h30m

Ingredients:
- ✓ 1 (10 pound) prime rib roast
- ✓ 10 cloves garlic, minced
- ✓ 2 tablespoons olive oil
- ✓ 2 teaspoons salt
- ✓ 2 teaspoons ground black pepper

✓ 2 teaspoons dried thyme

Directions: Put roast into a roasting pan, fatty side up. Combine thyme, pepper, salt, olive oil and garlic in a small bowl. Spread mixture atop the fatty layer of roast and leave roast to sit out for not more than 1 hour until it's at room temperature. Preheat an oven to 260 degrees C (500 degrees F). Bake roast for 20 minutes in the preheated oven, then decrease temperature to 165 degrees C (325 degrees F) and continue to roast for 60 to 75 more minutes. The internal temperature of the roast should read 57 degrees C (135 degrees F) for medium rare.

Leave the roast to rest for 10 or 15 minutes prior to carving so that meat can retain its juices.

GARLIC ROASTED SUMMER SQUASH

Serv.: 4| **Prep.:** 10m | **Cook:** 10m

Ingredients:
✓ 2 summer squash
✓ 1/4 cup olive oil
✓ 3 cloves garlic, minced, or more to taste
✓ 1 teaspoon herbes de Provence
✓ Salt to taste
✓ Ground black pepper to taste

Directions: Preheat an oven to 230°C/450°F. Trim squash ends; lengthwise, cut each squash in half. Crosswise, halve the halves again to get 4 pieces. Cut pieces in half 2 more times the long way to get 16 short pears from every squash. Toss garlic, olive oil and squash in bowl. Put in shallow baking dish. Sprinkle black pepper and salt. Roast squash for 5-10 minutes till garlic and spears begin to brown. After 5 minutes, check squash. Add time to avoid burning in 2-3-minute intervals.

GARLIC SALMON

Serv.: 6| **Prep.:** 15m | **Cook:** 25m

Ingredients:
✓ 1 1/2 pounds salmon fillet
✓ Salt and pepper to taste

✓ 3 cloves garlic, minced
✓ 1 sprig fresh dill, chopped
✓ 5 slices lemon
✓ 5 sprigs fresh dill weed
✓ 2 green onions, chopped

Directions: Preheat an oven to 230 degrees C (450 degrees F). Use cooking spray to spritz 2 large pieces of aluminum foil.

Put the salmon fillet onto one piece of foil. Drizzle the salmon using chopped dill, garlic, salt, and pepper. Spread slices of lemon slices over the fillet and then put a sprig of dill onto each lemon slice. Drizzle chopped scallions onto the fillet.

Use a second piece of foil to cover the salmon and then seal tightly by pinching the foil together. Transfer to a big baking dish or to baking sheet. Bake for 20 to 25 minutes in the oven until the salmon is flaked easily.

GARLICKY SUN DRIED TOMATO INFUSED OIL

Serv.: 32| **Prep.:** 10m | **Cook:** 0

Ingredients:
✓ 7 cloves garlic, chopped, or more to taste
✓ 10 sun-dried tomatoes, chopped
✓ 2 cups olive oil

Directions: Put sun-dried tomatoes and garlic into a 16-ounce dark glass bottle. With a funnel, pour olive oil into the bottle. Tightly close the bottle and chill in the fridge for 8 hours to overnight. Store the infused oil in the fridge.

GREEK FRIED CHICKEN

Serv.: 4| **Prep.:** 10m | **Cook:** 20m

Ingredients:
✓ 4 skinless chicken pieces
✓ 1/2 cup Greek olive oil
✓ 1 lemon, juiced
✓ 1 1/2 tablespoons freshly ground black pepper
✓ 1 teaspoon salt

- ✓ 1 1/2 tablespoons dried oregano
- ✓ 1 dash cinnamon
- ✓ 1 dash poultry seasoning
- ✓ 1/2 cup olive oil for frying
- ✓ 1 lemon, cut into wedges

Directions: Mix poultry seasoning, cinnamon, oregano, salt, pepper, lemon juice, 1/2 cup olive oil and chicken pieces in medium bowl; soak chicken for 5 minutes in seasonings and oil. Rub marinate in chicken with hands.

Heat 1/2 cup olive oil in 1 1/2-in. deep frying pan with lid to keep juices in chicken on low heat; lay chicken pieces carefully into frying pan. Put lid on pan; cook for 20 minutes till chicken is done, occasionally flipping pieces. Put heat on medium high; cook till outside of chicken browns.

Serve hot; use lemon wedges to garnish. For extra flavor, squeeze some lemon on chicken for delicious taste.

LEMON PEPPER CHICKEN

Serv.: 6| **Prep.:** 5m | **Cook:** 30m

Ingredients:
- ✓ 6 skinless, boneless chicken breast halves
- ✓ 1 teaspoon lemon pepper
- ✓ 1 pinch garlic powder
- ✓ 1 teaspoon onion powder

Directions: Preheat an oven to 175°C/350°F.
Put chicken into a 9x13-in. lightly greased baking dish; season to taste with onion powder, garlic powder and lemon pepper. In the preheated oven, bake for 15 minutes.
Flip chicken pieces; to taste, add more seasoning. Bake till juices are clear and chicken cooks through for 15 minutes more.

GRILLED SHRIMP AND SAUSAGES

Serv.: 8| **Prep.:** 10m | **Cook:** 10m

Ingredients:
Marinade:
- ✓ 2/3 cup extra-virgin olive oil

- ✓ 1 lemon, juiced
- ✓ 3 cloves garlic, chopped
- ✓ 2 tablespoons chopped Italian parsley
- ✓ 1/4 teaspoon red pepper flakes
- ✓ 1 pound shrimp, deveined, shells and tails on
- ✓ 1 pound Italian sausage, split open

Directions: In a big bowl, whisk red pepper flakes, parsley, garlic, lemon juice and oil. Add shrimp; marinade for 15 minutes.
Preheat the outdoor grill to medium high heat; oil grate lightly.
Take shrimp from marinade; shake excess off. Discard leftover marinade.
Cook sausage and shrimp on preheated grill for 10-15 minutes till cooked through.

GRILLED TEQUILA CILANTRO PINEAPPLE

Serv.: 4| **Prep.:** 10m | **Cook:** 10m

Ingredients:
- ✓ 1 fresh pineapple, peeled and cored
- ✓ 1 cup chopped fresh cilantro
- ✓ 1 cup tequila
- ✓ 1 1/2 tablespoons ground chipotle chiles
- ✓ 1 lemon
- ✓ 1 lime
- ✓ Salt and pepper to taste

Directions: Lengthwise, cut pineapple to 8 wedges. Put wedges into sealable plastic bag/container. Mix chipotle, tequila and cilantro in a small bowl. Put into container with pineapple. Cut lime and lemon in half. Squeeze some juice out; put fruit and juice into container. Season with pepper and salt.
Marinate for 1 hour minimum in the fridge, flipping pineapple once.
Preheat outdoor grill for medium high heat. Brush a light coat of oil on grate when coals are hot.
Grill wedges, 4-5 minutes per side. For sauce: Cook marinade on medium high heat in a saucepan; boil. Cook till sauce is syrupy and thick. It will be spicy.

GRILLED TOMATOES

Serv.: 16| Prep.: 15m | Cook: 10m

Ingredients:
- ✓ 8 tomatoes, halved lengthwise
- ✓ 1 tablespoon olive oil
- ✓ 2 cloves garlic, minced, or to taste
- ✓ 1 teaspoon salt and ground black pepper to taste

Directions: Preheat outdoor grill to medium high heat; oil grate lightly.
Drizzle olive oil on tomatoes cut sides. Sprinkle black pepper, salt and garlic.
On preheated grill, put tomatoes, cut sides up. Grill for 4 minutes or till it shows blackened grill marks and tomatoes begin to sizzle. Flip tomatoes. Grill for 3 more minutes till garlic is golden brown.

GRILLED TUNA

Serv.: 4| Prep.: 10m | Cook: 6m

Ingredients:
- ✓ 4 (6 ounce) albacore tuna steaks, 1 inch thick
- ✓ 3 tablespoons extra virgin olive oil
- ✓ Salt and ground black pepper to taste
- ✓ 1 lime, juiced
- ✓ 1/2 cup hickory wood chips, soaked

Directions: Mix olive oil and tuna steaks together in a big Ziplock bag. Seal the Ziplock bag and turn to coat the tuna steaks, keep in the fridge for an hour. Set the grill on medium heat and preheat. Once the coals are very hot, spread a handful of mesquite or hickory wood chips on top of the hot coals for flavor.
Lightly grease the grill grate. Put pepper and salt on the marinated tuna steak to taste and put on the preheated grill and grill for roughly 6 minutes, turn once to cook both sides. Put the grilled tuna steak on a serving plate and squeeze some fresh lime juice on top. Serve right away.

GRILLED TUNA SALAD

Serv.: 4| Prep.: 10m | Cook: 10m

Ingredients:
- ✓ 20 ounces fresh tuna steaks, 1 inch thick
- ✓ 3 tablespoons white wine
- ✓ 3 tablespoons olive oil
- ✓ 2 tablespoons red wine vinegar
- ✓ 1/2 teaspoon chopped fresh rosemary
- ✓ 1/2 teaspoon ground black pepper
- ✓ 1/8 teaspoon salt
- ✓ 1 clove garlic, minced
- ✓ 6 cups packed torn salad greens
- ✓ 1 cup halved cherry tomatoes

Directions: Preheat the grill for medium heat.
In a glass dish, add tuna. Mix garlic, salt, pepper, rosemary, red wine vinegar, olive oil and wine to prepare the vinaigrette. Add two tbsp. on top of fish and coat by flipping. Let it marinate for 15 - 30 minutes, flipping one time. Reserve leftover vinaigrette to make salad dressing.
Use cooking spray to coat grill rack and put on grill to heat for 60 seconds. Add tuna on grill 4 to 6 inches above hot coals. Use foil to tent or use lid to cover. Cook, flipping one time, just till tuna starts to flake easily when tested using a fork for about 7 minutes. Get rid of marinade.
Arrange salad greens among four dishes. Add hot tuna over greens and put in cherry tomatoes. Mix the leftover vinaigrette and sprinkle on top of salads.

GRILLED YELLOW SQUASH

Serv.: 8| Prep.: 10m | Cook: 20m

Ingredients:
- ✓ 4 medium yellow squash
- ✓ 1/2 cup extra virgin olive oil
- ✓ 2 cloves garlic, crushed
- ✓ Salt and pepper to taste

Directions: Preheat a grill to medium heat.

Horizontally, cut squash to 1/4-in. – 1/2-in. thick slices to get long strips that won't fall through grill. In a small pan, heat olive oil; add garlic cloves. Cook on medium heat till garlic is fragrant and starts to sizzle. Brush garlic oil on squash slices. Season with pepper and salt.

Grill squash slices till they reach desired tenderness or for 5-10 minutes per side. Brush with extra garlic oil. Occasionally turning to avoid burning or sticking.

CATFISH

Serv.: 4 | **Prep.:** 10m | **Cook:** 30m

Ingredients:
- ✓ 2 tablespoons cooking oil
- ✓ 1 onion, chopped
- ✓ 2 cloves garlic, crushed
- ✓ 4 (4 ounce) catfish fillets
- ✓ Salt and pepper to taste
- ✓ 1 1/2 cups coconut milk

Directions: In a skillet set on medium heat, add oil. Stir and cook the garlic and onion in the hot oil for 7-10 minutes until the garlic turns lightly browned and the onion is glossy. Add in the catfish; add pepper and salt to taste. Cook for 2 minutes, covered. Stir in the coconut milk; cook for approximately 10 minutes, covered, until the coconut milk looks oily.

GYROS

Serv.: 8 | **Prep.:** 20m | **Cook:** 1h15m

Ingredients:
- ✓ 1/4 cup chopped red onion
- ✓ 1 tablespoon minced garlic
- ✓ 1 tablespoon dried marjoram
- ✓ 1 tablespoon ground dried rosemary
- ✓ 2 teaspoons kosher salt
- ✓ 1/2 teaspoon freshly ground black pepper
- ✓ 1 pound 93%-lean ground beef
- ✓ 1 pound ground lamb

Directions: Start preheating the oven to 350°F (175°C).

In a food processor, process the red onion until it is minced finely. Put the onion into a piece of the cheesecloth; squeeze as much moisture from onion as you can. Put the onion back to the food processor. Put in garlic. Process until garlic is integrated well. Blend black pepper, kosher salt, rosemary and marjoram into onion mixture. Blend ground lamb and ground beef gradually with seasoning and onion mixture; alternately put in small amounts of each meat to mixture and process until well incorporated after each addition. Pack meat mixture firmly into the loaf pan, making sure no air pockets are trapped in meat.

Bake in prepared oven for 75 m or until no longer pink in middle. An instant-read thermometer should register at least 175°F (80°C) when inserted into middle. Drain the grease. Thinly slice to enjoy.

HERB GARLIC OIL

Serv.: 4 | **Prep.:** 5m | **Cook:** 1m

Ingredients:
- ✓ 1/2 cup olive oil
- ✓ 1 clove garlic, roughly chopped
- ✓ 1/4 cup extra-virgin olive oil (optional)
- ✓ 1/2 teaspoon basil
- ✓ 1/2 teaspoon oregano

Directions: Heat a skillet on medium-low heat. Pour olive oil slowly into the skillet, sliding skillet away from the burner if oil starts to splatter. Put in garlic, then cook for approximately 60 seconds until sizzling but now browned. Turn the heat off, leave the skillet on burner. Mix in oregano, basil and extra-virgin olive oil. Pour into a container and keep in the refrigerator for 8 hours to overnight, until flavors combined.

HERBED EGGPLANT SLICES

Serv.: 4 | **Prep.:** 15m | **Cook:** 15m

Ingredients:

- ✓ 1 clove garlic, minced
- ✓ 1 tablespoon minced fresh oregano
- ✓ 1/4 cup chopped fresh basil
- ✓ 1/2 cup chopped fresh parsley
- ✓ 1 eggplant, sliced into 1/2 inch rounds
- ✓ Salt to taste
- ✓ Ground black pepper to taste

Directions: Set oven to 205° C (400° F) and start preheating. Use cooking spray to coat a baking tray. Combine parsley, basil, oregano, and garlic in a small bowl. Mix thoroughly then put aside. Generously season pepper and salt on both sides of every eggplant slice. Transfer to the baking tray. Bake until tender and lightly browned, about 5-7 minutes per side. On eggplant slices, sprinkle herb mixture; broil 1/2 minute under the broiler. Remove to a serving plate; serve right away.

HERBED MUSHROOMS WITH WHITE WINE

Serv.: 6| **Prep.:** 10m | **Cook:** 15m

Ingredients:

- ✓ 1 tablespoon olive oil
- ✓ 1 1/2 pounds fresh mushrooms
- ✓ 1 teaspoon Italian seasoning
- ✓ 1/4 cup dry white wine
- ✓ 2 cloves garlic, minced
- ✓ Salt and pepper to taste
- ✓ 2 tablespoons chopped fresh chives

Directions: In a skillet, heat oil over medium heat and place the mushrooms, seasoning with Italian seasoning, and cook, stirring frequently, for 10 minutes.
Mix in the garlic and the wine, and continue to cook until most of the wine evaporates. Season with a sprinkle of chives, pepper, and salt, then continue to cook for 1 minute.

HERBED SALMON

Serv.: 4| **Prep.:** 10m | **Cook:** 20m

Ingredients:

- ✓ 2 pounds salmon
- ✓ 5 dried sage leaves
- ✓ 1 tablespoon dried thyme
- ✓ 1 pinch ground paprika
- ✓ 1 pinch ground cayenne pepper

Directions: Start preheating the oven to 350°F (175°C). Use cooking spray to spray a sheet of aluminum foil on one side. The aluminum foil must be big enough to wrap all around the salmon.
Put the fish on the oil-coated side of the foil. Use pepper, paprika, thyme, and sage to drizzle. Fold foil over the fish to enclose.
Put in the preheated oven and bake the salmon until a fork can easily flake it, about 20 minutes.

HERBED AND SPICED ROASTED BEEF TENDERLOIN

Serv.: 8| **Prep.:** 20m | **Cook:** 35m

Ingredients:

- ✓ 2 tablespoons fresh rosemary
- ✓ 2 tablespoons fresh thyme leaves
- ✓ 2 bay leaves
- ✓ 4 cloves garlic
- ✓ 1 large shallot, peeled and quartered
- ✓ 1 tablespoon grated orange zest
- ✓ 1 tablespoon coarse salt
- ✓ 1 teaspoon freshly ground black pepper
- ✓ 1/2 teaspoon ground nutmeg
- ✓ 1/4 teaspoon ground cloves
- ✓ 2 tablespoons olive oil
- ✓ 2 (2 pound) beef tenderloin roasts, trimmed

Directions: Put cloves, nutmeg, pepper, salt, orange zest, shallot, garlic, bay leaves, thyme and rosemary in a food processor. While adding oil, run machine; process till smooth. Evenly spread mixture on all tenderloin's sides; put beef into big glass baking dish. Use foil to cover; refrigerate for a minimum of 6 hours.
Preheat an oven to 200°C/400°F; put tenderloins onto rack in a big roasting pan.

In preheated oven, roast beef for 35 minutes till inserted meat thermometer in middle of beef reads 140°. Remove from oven; loosely cover with foil and allow to stand about 10 minutes. Cut beef; serve.

INSTANT POT® BONE BROTH

Serv.: 6 | **Prep.:** 10m | **Cook:** 2h10m

Ingredients:
- ✓ 1 chicken carcass
- ✓ 2 carrots, cut in chunks
- ✓ 1 cup chopped celery
- ✓ 1 tablespoon apple cider vinegar
- ✓ 2 teaspoons ground turmeric
- ✓ 3 cloves garlic
- ✓ 1 teaspoon minced fresh ginger root
- ✓ 4 cups warm water, or as needed

Directions: On an Instant Pot® or any multi-functional pressure cooker, mix chicken carcass, celery, carrots, garlic, ginger, turmeric and vinegar. Pour enough water to cover the vegetables and bones in the pot. Close and secure the lid and adjust setting to Manual. Set the timer to 120 minutes. Let the pressure build for 10 to 15 minutes.
Follow manufacturer's direction in using natural-release method and let the pressure go, 10 to 40 minutes. Unseal and remove cover for the broth to cool slightly. Use a fine metal sieve to remove the vegetables and all the bits of bones.

INSTANT POT® EGG SHAKSHUKA WITH KALE

Serv.: 4 | **Prep.:** 10m | **Cook:** 15m

Ingredients:
- ✓ 1 tablespoon olive oil
- ✓ 1/2 onion, diced
- ✓ 1/2 red bell pepper, diced
- ✓ 2 cloves garlic, minced
- ✓ 1 teaspoon chili powder
- ✓ 1/2 teaspoon smoked paprika
- ✓ 1/2 teaspoon ground cumin
- ✓ 2 cups baby kale
- ✓ 1 1/2 cups marinara sauce
- ✓ 1/2 teaspoon sea salt
- ✓ 1/2 teaspoon ground black pepper
- ✓ 4 eggs
- ✓ 1 tablespoon chopped fresh parsley

Directions: Set the multi-functional pressure cooker on Sauté mode. Pour olive oil in and heat. Add the cumin, onion, paprika, red bell pepper, chili powder, and garlic; cook for 3 minutes until soft. Stir in kale and cook for another 2 minutes until soft. Mix in the marinara sauce, season with pepper and salt. Turn off heat; cool for 5 minutes Carefully break eggs in the pot, space it evenly. Close then lock the lid and set the pressure to low and the timer to 0 minutes as specified in the manufacturer's manual. When it beeps, use the quick-release method to relieve the pressure following the cooker's manual for 2 minutes. Uncover and take out lid. Garnish with parsley.

INSTANT TOMATO CHUTNEY

Serv.: 8 | **Prep.:** 5m | **Cook:** 3m

Ingredients:
- ✓ 4 large ripe tomatoes, chopped
- ✓ 2 teaspoons dry mustard powder
- ✓ 1 teaspoon ground turmeric
- ✓ 2 cloves garlic, peeled (optional)
- ✓ 1 teaspoon fenugreek seeds
- ✓ 2 dried red chile peppers
- ✓ 2 teaspoons salt
- ✓ 1 teaspoon vegetable oil
- ✓ 1 teaspoon chili powder (optional)

Directions: Mix together chili powder, oil, salt, chilies, fenugreek, garlic, turmeric, mustard powder and the tomatoes in a microwave-safe dish. Cook on high power until the tomatoes are hot and wilted, or about 3 minutes. Discard dried chilies and the garlic cloves, stir well and serve.

Coconut and Sweet Potato Mash

Serv.: 4| **Prep.:** 12m | **Cook:** 10m

Ingredients:
- 3 sweet potatoes
- 1 small lime, juiced
- 1 green onion, finely chopped
- 1 teaspoon ground cumin
- 1/2 teaspoon salt
- 1/4 teaspoon ground cinnamon
- 1/4 teaspoon pepper
- 1 1/2 cups Gay Lea Real Coconut Whipped Cream

Directions: Use a fork or paring knife to pierce sweet potatoes for a couple of times. Microwave about 10-12 minutes on high setting, or until very tender. Cool just enough to handle easily.
Scrape potato flesh from skins into a bowl and get rid of skins. Use a fork to mash well, then stir in pepper, cinnamon, salt, cumin, onion and lime juice. Fold into the sweet potato mixture with coconut whipped cream until blended. Serve promptly.

Italian Kale

Serv.: 4| **Prep.:** 5m | **Cook:** 15m

Ingredients:
- 1 bunch kale, stems removed and leaves coarsely chopped
- 1 clove garlic, minced
- 1 tablespoon olive oil
- 2 tablespoons balsamic vinegar
- Salt and ground black pepper to taste

Directions: In a big saucepan, cook the kale with a cover on medium high heat, until kale leaves are wilted. When the volume of kale is decreased by half, take off the cover then stir in vinegar, olive oil and garlic. Cook and stir for 2 minutes longer, then put in pepper and salt to taste.

Kale Garlic Saute

Serv.: 6| **Prep.:** 10m | **Cook:** 20m

Ingredients:
- 6 slices bacon
- 1 onion, chopped
- 1 bunch kale, stemmed and chopped
- 6 cloves garlic, minced
- 2 ounces cashews, or to taste
- 1 teaspoon rice vinegar, or to taste

Directions: In a big skillet, add bacon and cook on moderately high heat for 10 minutes, while turning sometimes, until browned evenly. Turn the bacon slices onto paper towels to drain and save 1 tbsp. bacon grease in the skillet.
In the bacon grease, cook and stir onion on moderate heat for 5-10 minutes, until softened.
Put in kale then cook and stir for 2-3 minutes, until wilted a little bit. Stir into kale mixture with garlic and cook for 1 minute, until garlic is tangy.
Turn kale mixture to a serving bowl. Crumble bacon, dust cashews and drizzle rice vinegar over kale.

Kale Orange Banana Smoothie

Serv.: 1| **Prep.:** 10m | **Cook:** 0

Ingredients:
- 1 orange, peeled
- 1/2 cup water
- 1 leaf kale, torn into several pieces
- 2 ripe bananas, peeled

Directions: In a blender, put in the orange and blend until most part is juice.
Add in kale and water and blend on High speed until the kale liquefies.
Blend in banana chunks on low speed until well combined. Turn to high speed until the texture resembles a pudding.

KALE SALAD WITH POMEGRANATE, SUNFLOWER SEEDS

Serv.: 6| **Prep.:** 20m | **Cook:** 0

Ingredients:
- ✓ 1/2 pound kale
- ✓ 1 1/2 cups pomegranate seeds
- ✓ 2 tablespoons sunflower seeds
- ✓ 1/3 cup sliced almonds
- ✓ 5 tablespoons red pepper seasoned rice vinegar
- ✓ 5 tablespoons balsamic vinegar
- ✓ 3 tablespoons extra virgin olive oil
- ✓ Salt to taste

Directions: Wash and drain off the excess water from the kale. Throw away the stems and center ribs. Roughly chop the leaves to get a fine yet still quite leafy appearance. Toss the sliced almonds, sunflower seeds, pomegranate seeds and chopped kale together in a large bowl. Combine by tossing. Continue tossing after adding the olive oil, balsamic vinegar and rice vinegar over the kale mixture. Add salt to finish it off.

KALE WITH CARAMELIZED ONIONS

Serv.: 4| **Prep.:** 10m | **Cook:** 45m

Ingredients:
- ✓ 2 tablespoons olive oil
- ✓ 1/2 onion, halved and thinly sliced
- ✓ 3 cloves garlic, minced
- ✓ 1 bunch curly kale, stemmed and coarsely chopped
- ✓ 2 cups water
- ✓ Salt and ground black pepper to taste
- ✓ 1 tablespoon balsamic vinegar
- ✓ 1/3 cup chopped almonds

Directions: In a heavy pot or a Dutch oven over medium heat, heat oil; cook while stirring onion till softened and starting to brown, about 10-15 minutes. Put garlic into onion; cook while stirring for around 1 minute; till aromatic.

Mix water and kale into the onion mixture. Cook with a cover in a Dutch oven for around 30 minutes, till kale is tender; season with pepper and salt. Sprinkle caramelized onions and kale with balsamic vinegar; top with almonds.

KALE WITH KIWI

Serv.: 2| **Prep.:** 20m | **Cook:** 10m

Ingredients:
- ✓ 2 teaspoons coconut oil
- ✓ 2 cloves garlic, chopped
- ✓ 1 teaspoon minced fresh ginger
- ✓ 1/4 teaspoon sea salt
- ✓ 1/2 teaspoon freshly ground black pepper
- ✓ 2 kiwis, peeled and coarsely chopped
- ✓ 1 tablespoon fresh oregano leaves
- ✓ 1 bunch lacinato (dinosaur) kale, washed and sliced thin
- ✓ 2 tablespoons blanched slivered almonds

Directions: Pour coconut oil in a pan and heat over medium-high heat. Mixed in sliced ginger and garlic, and season with freshly-ground pepper and sea salt; cook and stir for about 3 minutes, until the garlic changes color. Add oregano leaves and chopped kiwi and cook for another 2 minutes. Stir in kale; lower the heat to medium and let cook for about 5 minutes until the kale becomes tender and turns into a dark green color. Top with thinly-sliced almonds and season to taste.

LEMON CHICKEN WITH BROCCOLI

Serv.: 4| **Prep.:** 20m | **Cook:** 40m

Ingredients:
- ✓ 1 large lemon
- ✓ 2 tablespoons olive oil
- ✓ 3 pounds chicken parts
- ✓ 1 medium onion, diced
- ✓ 1 clove garlic, minced
- ✓ 2 packets Swanson® Flavor Boost™ Concentrated Chicken Broth
- ✓ 3 cups fresh broccoli florets

Directions: Squeeze 1/4 cup juice from the lemon and grate 1 tablespoon zest.

Put 1 tablespoon oil and heat over medium-high heat in a 12-inch skillet. Put in the chicken and cook until all sides are browned well. Take the chicken from the skillet. Discard any fat.

Lower the heat to medium. Put the rest of the oil in the skillet. Place in the garlic and onion and stir and cook for 2 minutes. Mix in the lemon juice and concentrated broth. Put the chicken back to the skillet. Lower the heat to low. Cook for 20 minutes, covered, or until chicken is cooked through.

Mix the lemon zest and broccoli in the skillet. Cook, covered until the broccoli turns tender-crisp.

LEMON COCONUT CLEANSER

Serv.: 2| **Prep.:** 10m | **Cook:** 0

Ingredients:
- ✓ 1 cup frozen mango chunks
- ✓ 1/2 lemon, peeled
- ✓ 1 cup fresh spinach
- ✓ 1/4 unpeeled zucchini, chopped
- ✓ 3/4 cup water
- ✓ 4 ice cubes, or more to taste
- ✓ 1 tablespoon coconut oil, melted

Directions: In a high-speed blender, mix coconut oil, mango chunks, ice cubes, lemon, water, spinach, and zucchini together until the mixture is smooth.

LEMON ROSEMARY SALMON

Serv.: 2| **Prep.:** 10m | **Cook:** 20m

Ingredients:
- ✓ 1 lemon, thinly sliced
- ✓ 4 sprigs fresh rosemary
- ✓ 2 salmon fillets, bones and skin removed
- ✓ Salt to taste
- ✓ 1 tablespoon olive oil, or as needed

Directions: Preheat the oven to 200 degrees C (400 degrees F).

Lay out half the lemon slices in a single layer in a baking dish. Layer with two sprigs rosemary and place salmon fillets on top. Sprinkle the salmon with salt, spread a layer of the remaining rosemary sprigs and place the remaining lemon slices on top. Trickle with olive oil.

Bake for 20 minutes in the oven or until the fish flakes easily with a fork.

MANGO CHERRY SMOOTHIE

Serv.: 2| **Prep.:** 10m | **Cook:** 0

Ingredients:
- ✓ 2 cups pitted cherries
- ✓ 1 cup chopped mango
- ✓ 1 cup water
- ✓ 1 cup ice cubes

Directions: Use a blender to blend together ice cubes, water, mango, and cherries until smooth.

MANGO MADNESS SALAD

Serv.: 12 | **Prep.:** 20m | **Cook:** 0

Ingredients:
- ✓ 5 mango, peeled and diced
- ✓ 6 fresh strawberries, sliced
- ✓ 1/2 cup blackberries
- ✓ 1/4 cup chopped cilantro
- ✓ 1/2 lime, juiced

Directions: In a bowl, combine blackberries, strawberries and mangos. Toss lime and cilantro. Put in the fridge for 60 minutes.

MANGO PAPAYA SALSA

Serv.: 8| **Prep.:** 15m | **Cook:**

Ingredients:
- ✓ 1 mango - peeled, seeded and diced
- ✓ 1 papaya - peeled, seeded and diced
- ✓ 1 large red bell pepper, seeded and diced
- ✓ 1 avocado - peeled, pitted and diced
- ✓ 1/2 sweet onion, peeled and diced

✓ 2 tablespoons chopped fresh cilantro
✓ 2 tablespoons balsamic vinegar
✓ Salt and pepper to taste

Directions: Combine in a medium bowl the balsamic vinegar, cilantro, sweet onion, avocado, red bell pepper, papaya and mango. Add pepper and salt to taste. Then cover and refrigerate for at least 30 minutes until chilled then serve.

MANGO PINEAPPLE SALAD WITH MINT

Serv.: 6| **Prep.:** 20m | **Cook:** 0

Ingredients:
✓ 2 cups peeled, diced ripe mango
✓ 1 cup chopped fresh pineapple
✓ 1/4 cup dried cranberries
✓ 1/4 cup flaked coconut
✓ 1/4 sprig chopped fresh mint

Directions: Mix coconut, cranberries, pineapple and mango together in a medium bowl. Top with mint for decoration. Cover and place in the fridge until ready to serve.

MANGO TANGO

Serv.: 2| **Prep.:** 10m | **Cook:** 0

Ingredients:
✓ 2 medium mangos, peeled and sliced
✓ 2 peeled limes
✓ 2 apples, cored and quartered

Directions: In a juice machine, juice apples, limes and mango, then serve over ice.

MANGO BACON BUTTERNUT SQUASH

Serv.: 2| **Prep.:** 10m | **Cook:** 25m

Ingredients:
✓ 3 slices bacon, cut into 1/4-inch squares
✓ 1 butternut squash, peeled and cubed
✓ 1 teaspoon thyme
✓ 1 mango, peeled and cubed

✓ Salt and ground black pepper, to taste

Directions: Put bacon in a large frying pan and cook over medium-high heat power, turning from time to time, until evenly browned, for about 5 minutes. Put in thyme and squash; cook and stir until squash begins to brown, about 10 to 15 minutes. Put the mango; cook and stir until heated thoroughly, for about 5 minutes.

MANGU

Serv.: 6| **Prep.:** 15m | **Cook:** 25m

Ingredients:
✓ 3 green plantains
✓ 1 quart water
✓ 1/4 cup olive oil
✓ 1 cup sliced white onion
✓ 1 1/2 tablespoons salt
✓ 1 cup sliced Anaheim peppers

Directions: In a saucepan, put water and plantains. Boil, and cook for 20 minutes, till plantains are soft yet slightly firm. Drain, setting aside a cup of liquid. Allow plantains to cool, and take off skin.
In a skillet over medium heat, heat olive oil, and sauté onion till soft.
Mash plantains along with salt and reserved liquid in a bowl. Move to a food processor, stir in peppers, and puree. Serve pureed plantain mixture with onions on top.

MANTECA FRIED CARNITAS

Serv.: 20| **Prep.:** 15m | **Cook:** 1h

Ingredients:
✓ 1 gallon lard for frying
✓ 5 pounds boneless pork shoulder, cut into 1 1/2-inch cubes
✓ 6 bay leaves
✓ 2 tablespoons kosher salt
✓ 1 1/2 teaspoons coarse ground black pepper
✓ 2 large onions, quartered
✓ 3 whole garlic cloves
✓ 1 large orange, halved

Directions: Heat lard in deep roasting pan on medium heat; mix garlic, onions, pepper, salt, bay leaves and pork in. Squeeze orange into mixture; drop orange halves in. if needed, add extra lard to cover all ingredients.

Cook for 45-60 minutes till pork is tender enough to shred with fork. Discard garlic, onion and orange; use slotted spoon to strain pork cubes from lard.

MICROWAVE PEACH PLUM BUTTER

Serv.: 16 | **Prep.:** 10m | **Cook:** 15m

Ingredients:
- ✓ 1 cup finely chopped, peeled peaches
- ✓ 1 cup pitted, chopped plums
- ✓ 1 tablespoon water
- ✓ 1/2 teaspoon ground cinnamon
- ✓ 1/2 teaspoon ground ginger
- ✓ 1/2 cup granular no-calorie sucralose sweetener (such as Splenda®)

Directions: In a microwavable ceramic or glass bowl, mix water, plums and peaches. In microwave, heat on high in 3-minute intervals for 15 minutes, mixing every after heating, till mixture is really thick. Mix in sweetener, ginger and cinnamon. Into a jar, put the fruit butter. Place cover and chill till set to use.

PORK WITH OLIVE

Serv.: 2 | **Prep.:** 30m | **Cook:** 20m

Ingredients:
- ✓ 2 tablespoons olive oil
- ✓ 1/2 pound pork loin, sliced and cut into thin strips
- ✓ 1/2 red bell pepper, chopped
- ✓ 1/2 yellow bell pepper, chopped
- ✓ 1/2 green bell pepper, chopped
- ✓ 1 carrot, peeled and chopped
- ✓ 5 Brussels sprouts, trimmed and chopped
- ✓ 4 cloves garlic, minced
- ✓ 1/4 cup white onion, chopped
- ✓ 4 sprigs Italian flat leaf parsley, chopped
- ✓ 3 stalks celery, chopped
- ✓ 2 (1/2 inch) pieces fresh ginger root, finely chopped
- ✓ 1/2 (8 ounce) can water chestnuts, drained and chopped
- ✓ 2 sprigs fresh mint, chopped

Directions: Pour in the olive oil into a big skillet and warm it up at medium high heat. Insert the pork strips, frying until it starts browning. Insert Brussels sprouts, carrot, green, yellow and red bell peppers, tossing with oil until well coated. Add enough water to ensure the pan's base is coated, cooking for around 5 minutes until the peppers start softening. During the process, stir regularly. Adjust the heat setting to medium before adding the celery, parsley, onion and garlic, stirring. Leave it simmering for 5-7 minutes. Insert ginger then leave it simmering for several extra minutes. Add mint and water chestnuts, stirring. Leave it simmering until flavors are combined, about 2-3 minutes. Serve right away.

MOIST GARLIC ROASTED CHICKEN

Serv.: 6 | **Prep.:** 15m | **Cook:** 1h30m

Ingredients:
- ✓ 1 (4 pound) whole chicken
- ✓ Salt and pepper to taste
- ✓ 1 large lemon, sliced
- ✓ 6 cloves garlic, sliced
- ✓ 6 sprigs thyme

Directions: Start preheating the oven to 325°F (165°C).

In the center of a roasting tray, add a big parchment paper sheet. The parchment must be big enough to fully wrap the chicken. Use pepper and salt to season the chicken, stuff 1/2 of the lemon slices in, and put the breast side up in the center of the parchment paper. Evenly sprinkle over the chicken with thyme sprigs and garlic slices. Place over the breast with the leftover lemon slices. Make a loose package with the parchment fold over the chicken.

Put in the preheated oven and bake for 1 1/2-2 hours until the chicken has cooked. A meat thermometer should register 180°F when you insert one into the thickest section of the thigh.

Molasses Glazed Sweet Potatoes with Sage Pecans

Serv.: 6| **Prep.:** 10m | **Cook:** 35m

Ingredients:
- ✓ 4 large sweet potatoes, peeled and cut into 1-inch cubes
- ✓ 6 tablespoons Crisco® Pure Canola Oil, divided
- ✓ 15 fresh sage leaves
- ✓ 1/3 cup molasses
- ✓ 1/4 teaspoon ground cinnamon
- ✓ 1/8 teaspoon ground red pepper
- ✓ Salt to taste
- ✓ 1/3 cup coarsely chopped pecans

Directions: Heat an oven to 375 °F. Line foil on 2 baking sheets. Coat the sweet potatoes with 3 tbsp. of oil. Put on prepped baking sheets. Bake till easily pierced with fork for 28 to 32 minutes.
In a big skillet, heat the leftover 3 tablespoons of oil over medium-high heat. Put in the sage leaves. Cook till edges starts to brown for 1 to 2 minutes. Take out using a slotted spoon.
To skillet, put the sweet potatoes. Cook over medium-high heat for 2 minutes. Put in red pepper, cinnamon and molasses. Cook, mixing from time to time, for 2 to 3 minutes till molasses become thick. Add salt to season. Put in a serving dish. Place pecans and crumbled sage leaves on top.

Kimchi Eggs

Serv.: 2| **Prep.:** 5m | **Cook:** 5m

Ingredients:
- ✓ 2 tablespoons vegetable oil
- ✓ 1 cup kimchi, or to taste
- ✓ 2 large eggs, beaten

Directions: Over medium heat, heat oil in a wok or skillet and then cook kimchi in the hot oil for about

2 minutes until softened. Place in the eggs. Cook while stirring the kimchi and eggs for 2 to 3 minutes until eggs are set.

European Sausage Patties

Serv.: 8| **Prep.:** 5m | **Cook:** 15m

Ingredients:
- ✓ 2 pounds ground turkey
- ✓ 3/4 teaspoon ground ginger
- ✓ 1 1/2 teaspoons salt
- ✓ 1 teaspoon dried sage
- ✓ 1/4 teaspoon cayenne pepper
- ✓ 1 1/2 teaspoons ground black pepper

Directions: In a big bowl, combine black pepper, cayenne pepper, sage, salt, ginger and ground turkey till well-blended.
Heat a skillet on medium high heat, and coat using the non-stick cooking spray. Shape turkey sausage into patties, and fry till becoming brown on both sides and not pink in middle anymore. This process should take roughly 15 minutes.

Greek Octopus in Tomato Sauce

Serv.: 6| **Prep.:** 20m | **Cook:** 1h10m

Ingredients:
- ✓ 2 pounds octopus, cut into 3-inch pieces
- ✓ 3/4 cup olive oil
- ✓ 8 small red onions, cut into thin wedges
- ✓ 3 bay leaves
- ✓ 2 cups crushed tomatoes
- ✓ 1/2 teaspoon sea salt
- ✓ Freshly ground black pepper to taste

Directions: In a big saucepan, put octopus pieces. Cover then cook for 10-15 minutes on medium-high heat until the octopus releases its juices. Take out cover; keep simmering for 20-25 minutes until liquid reduces to 3-4 tablespoons.
Drizzle olive oil on octopus. Mix in bay leaves and onions. Sauté for about 10 minutes until onions are soft. Add pepper, salt, and tomatoes. Lower heat to medium-low. Cover then simmer for about 25

minutes until sauce is thick and octopus is tender. Cook uncovered in the final 10 minutes if sauce is thin.

FILLET ARCTIC CHAR WITH LIME

Serv.: 2| **Prep.:** 10m | **Cook:** 15m

Ingredients:
- ✓ 1 (10 ounce) fillet arctic char, rinsed and patted dry
- ✓ 1 pinch sea salt to taste
- ✓ 1 lime, zested and juiced
- ✓ 1/4 cup olive oil
- ✓ 1/4 cup sherry wine
- ✓ 3 sprigs rosemary, leaves stripped
- ✓ 2 cloves garlic
- ✓ Ground black pepper to taste
- ✓ 1 teaspoon cayenne pepper, or to taste

Directions: Set the oven to 200°C (400°F) to preheat. Line aluminum foil on a baking dish.
Season salt on arctic char, then put in the lined baking dish. Top with lime zest.
In a food processor, mix garlic, rosemary, sherry, olive oil, and lime juice; pulse until finely chopped. Spread over fish with the mixture and season with cayenne pepper and black pepper.
Put in the preheated oven and bake for 12-15 minutes, until fish easily flakes with a fork, using pan juices to baste halfway through. When fish is nearly being cooked, switch oven to broil until browned, about remaining 2 minutes.

OKRA AND TOMATOES

Serv.: 6| **Prep.:** 10m | **Cook:** 20m

Ingredients:
- ✓ 2 slices bacon
- ✓ 1 pound frozen okra, thawed and sliced
- ✓ 1 small onion, chopped
- ✓ 1/2 green bell pepper, chopped
- ✓ 2 celery, chopped
- ✓ 1 (14.5 ounce) can stewed tomatoes
- ✓ Salt and pepper to taste

Directions: In a big, deep skillet, put the bacon in. Over medium-high heat, cook until it turns brown evenly. Once done, drain and crumble the bacon. Set aside.
Remove the bacon from the pan. In the same pan, sauté the celery, pepper, onion and the okra until tender. Put the pepper, salt and tomatoes. Cook until the tomatoes are heated through.
If desired, garnish with the crumbled bacon.

OKRA WITH TOMATOES

Serv.: 6| **Prep.:** 15m | **Cook:** 15m

Ingredients:
- ✓ 1 teaspoon olive oil
- ✓ 3 cloves garlic, minced
- ✓ 1 small onion, minced
- ✓ 1 teaspoon cayenne pepper
- ✓ 1/2 green bell pepper, minced
- ✓ 1 pound frozen sliced okra
- ✓ 1 (8 ounce) can canned diced tomatoes
- ✓ 1 (15 ounce) can stewed tomatoes
- ✓ Salt and ground black pepper to taste

Directions: Over medium heat, put the skillet with the olive oil, enough to cover the bottom of the skillet. Put the cayenne pepper, onion and the garlic. Stir until it is fragrant. Mix the green pepper. For about 5 minutes, stir and cook until it is tender. Mix the frozen okra. Wait for 5 more minutes to allow to cook. Mix the stewed and the diced tomatoes and season with pepper and salt. Turn the heat to medium low. Let it simmer for 5-7 minutes until all the vegetables are tender.

OLIVE OIL DIPPING SAUCE

Serv.: 16| **Prep.:** 5m | **Cook:** 5m

Ingredients:
- ✓ 1 cup extra-virgin olive oil
- ✓ 2 cloves garlic, minced
- ✓ 1/4 teaspoon dried oregano
- ✓ 1 pinch salt, or to taste
- ✓ 1 pinch dried rosemary, or to taste

- ✓ 1 pinch dried basil, or to taste
- ✓ Ground black pepper to taste

Directions: In a skillet, mix together pepper, basil, rosemary, salt, oregano, garlic and olive oil over medium heat; cook for 5 minutes until the garlic starts sizzling. Take it off the heat immediately.

OMELET MUFFINS WITH KALE AND BROCCOLI

Serv.: 12| **Prep.:** 20m | **Cook:** 20m

Ingredients:
- ✓ 8 eggs
- ✓ 2 tablespoons heavy whipping cream
- ✓ 1/4 teaspoon salt
- ✓ 1/4 teaspoon ground black pepper
- ✓ 1 cup finely chopped kale
- ✓ 1/2 cup finely chopped broccoli
- ✓ 1/4 cup diced onion
- ✓ 1/2 cup shredded Cheddar cheese

Directions: Set an oven to 175°C (350°F) and start preheating. Use paper liners to line a muffin tin.
In a bowl, whisk pepper, salt, heavy cream, and eggs using an electric mixer. Fold in onion, broccoli, and kale until combined evenly. Add the mixture into the lined muffin tin, stuffing each cup to 3/4 full.
In the prepared oven, bake for 20-25 minutes until a toothpick comes out without resistance when inserted into the center.
Melt the cheese atop muffins, then serve.

ONION PEPPER RELISH

Serv.: 86| **Prep.:** 10m | **Cook:** 15m

Ingredients:
- ✓ 10 large yellow onions, cut into wedges
- ✓ 15 fresh jalapeno peppers
- ✓ 3 cups white vinegar
- ✓ 2 tablespoons cracked black pepper
- ✓ 2 tablespoons pickling salt

Directions: In a food processor, using a shredding blade, shred the jalapeno peppers and onions.
In a large pot, mix the black pepper, onion, salt, jalapeno pepper, and vinegar. Bring the mixture to a full boil over medium heat while stirring the mixture often. Let it cook for 10 minutes.
Fill the sterilized pint canning jars firmly with the mixture, filling it up to 3/4-inch of the top. Drizzle cooking liquid all over the onions, filling it up to 1/2 inch of the top. Use a spatula to stir the mixture gently and to remove all of the air bubbles. Use a clean damp cloth to wipe the rims of the jars.
Adjust the lids and rings tightly. Place the jars in a boiling water bath and process them for 5 minutes.

ONION SALMON

Serv.: 4| **Prep.:** 10m | **Cook:** 15m

Ingredients:
- ✓ 1 pound salmon fillet
- ✓ 1 onion, sliced into rings
- ✓ Freshly ground black pepper

Directions: Start preheating an outdoor grill to medium heat and lightly grease the grate.
On a big sheet of aluminum foil, put salmon. Top the fillets with onion rings. Season with pepper. Fold the foil around the salmon, do not close the top.
Put the salmon (still in the foil) onto the preheated grill and shut the lid. Cook until the fish is flaky with a fork, about 15 minutes.

ORANGE ROMAINE SALAD

Serv.: 8| **Prep.:** | **Cook:**

Ingredients:
- ✓ 1/4 cup red wine vinegar
- ✓ 3/4 cup vegetable oil
- ✓ 1 tablespoon honey
- ✓ 1/2 teaspoon salt
- ✓ 1/4 teaspoon ground black pepper
- ✓ 1/4 cup chopped green onion

✓ 1 large head romaine lettuce, torn into bite-size pieces
✓ 3 oranges, peeled and thinly sliced

Directions: Add green onion, pepper, salt, honey, oil and vinegar into a small container with a tight-fitting lid. Close the lid and shake it as hard as possible to get everything well incorporated.
In a large serving bowl, add in the romaine lettuce. Toss it with the dressing. Do another gentle toss after adding the orange slices. Serve instantly.

ORANGE SALMON

Serv.: 2| **Prep.:** 15m | **Cook:** 25m

Ingredients:
✓ 2 blood oranges, peeled and sliced into rounds
✓ 1 pound salmon fillets
✓ 1/2 teaspoon freshly grated nutmeg
✓ 1 cup red wine

Directions: Heat oven to 175°C (350°F) beforehand. In the bottom of a medium baking dish, place orange slices in a single layer. Lay salmon on oranges and use nutmeg to dredge it with. Over the salmon, add red wine.
In the preheated oven, cover and allow to bake for 20 to 25 minutes till easily flakes with a fork.

ORANGE SALMON WITH CREOLE SEASONING

Serv.: 2| **Prep.:** 10m | **Cook:** 10m

Ingredients:
✓ 1 tablespoon vegetable oil
✓ 2 salmon steaks
✓ 1 tablespoon Creole seasoning, or to taste
✓ 1 orange, juiced

Directions: Heat oil over medium in a skillet. Sprinkle Creole seasoning over salmon to season. Cook fish in heated oil until golden brown, about 2 to 3 minutes per side.

Turn heat to low, pour in orange juice. Keep cooking until fish is fork-tender, or about 5 minutes.

OSSO BUCCO STYLE BEEF SHANK

Serv.: 2| **Prep.:** 10m | **Cook:** 1h50m

Ingredients:
✓ 2 tablespoons olive oil
✓ 1 onion, chopped
✓ 3 cloves garlic, chopped
✓ 1 pound beef shank
✓ 1/4 teaspoon dried thyme
✓ 1/4 teaspoon dried oregano
✓ 1/4 teaspoon dried rosemary
✓ 1/4 teaspoon dried marjoram
✓ 1 (16 ounce) can diced tomatoes
✓ 1 (6 ounce) can tomato paste
✓ water
✓ 1 tablespoon lemon zest
✓ 1 teaspoon sea salt
✓ 1/2 teaspoon coarsely ground black pepper

Directions: Put the olive oil in a big saucepan and let it heat up over medium heat setting. Put in the garlic and onion and sauté it for about 5 minutes until it is tender. Place the sautéed garlic and onion onto a plate.
Adjust the heat to medium-high setting. Put in the beef shank and let it cook for about 5 minutes on every side until it turns brown in color. Put the sautéed garlic and onion back into the pan. Season the beef mixture with rosemary, thyme, marjoram and oregano to taste.
Put the tomato paste and tomatoes into the same saucepan. Pour water into the empty tomato paste can to get any remaining tomato paste from the can then pour it into the mixture.
Add in the salt, black pepper and lemon zest and give it a mix.
Let the mixture boil then lower the heat to low setting; cover the pan and let the mixture simmer for 1 1/2 to 2 hours until the beef is really tender.

OVEN BAKED SWAI

Serv.: 2| **Prep.:** 10m | **Cook:** 35m

Ingredients:
- ✓ 2 (4 ounce) fillets swai fish
- ✓ Salt and ground black pepper to taste
- ✓ 1 tablespoon olive oil, or as needed
- ✓ 1 onion, chopped
- ✓ 1 clove garlic, minced
- ✓ 1 (14.5 ounce) can petite diced tomatoes

Directions: Turn oven to 400°F (200°C) to preheat. Arrange swai fish in a glass casserole dish; sprinkle with black pepper and salt to season.
Heat olive oil over medium heat in a large skillet; cook and mix onion for about 10 minutes until tender. Add garlic; cook for about 1 minutes until aromatic. Add tomatoes over the top of onion mixture in the skillet; cook while mixing for about 5 minutes until thoroughly heated. Scoop tomato mixture all over the fish.
Bake for about 20 minutes in the preheated oven until fish is fork-tender.

OVEN ROASTED GRAPE TOMATOES

Serv.: 2| **Prep.:** 15m | **Cook:** 30m

Ingredients:
- ✓ 1 pound grape tomatoes, halved
- ✓ 1 tablespoon olive oil
- ✓ 2 cloves garlic, minced
- ✓ 5 fresh basil leaves, chopped
- ✓ 1 teaspoon chopped fresh thyme
- ✓ Salt to taste

Directions: Preheat the oven to 175°C or 350°F.
In a big square of aluminum foil, put the tomatoes. Sprinkle olive oil on tomatoes and put salt, thyme, basil and garlic on top. Wrap tomato mixture with foil securing tightly to retain juices inside.
In the preheated oven, bake for about half an hour till tomatoes are soft. Slightly cool.

OVEN BAKED BANANA CHIPS

Serv.: 1| **Prep.:** 5m | **Cook:** 0

Ingredients:
- ✓ 1 firm banana, thinly sliced

Directions: Prepare oven by heating to 80° C or 175° F. Place parchment paper on a baking sheet. Arrange banana slices in one layer on the prepared baking sheet.
Bake for 1 hour in the oven. Flip banana slices. Bake for another hour until crisp and dry.

PALEO BAKED EGGS IN AVOCADO

Serv.: 2| **Prep.:** 10m | **Cook:** 15m

Ingredients:
- ✓ 2 small eggs
- ✓ 1 avocado, halved and pitted
- ✓ 2 slices cooked bacon, crumbled
- ✓ 2 teaspoons chopped fresh chives, or to taste
- ✓ 1 pinch dried parsley, or to taste
- ✓ 1 pinch sea salt and ground black pepper to taste

Directions: Set the oven to 220°C or 425°F to preheat.
Crack into a bowl with eggs and make sure to keep the yolks intact.
In a baking dish, arrange avocado halves and rest them along the edge to make sure avocado will not tip over. Scoop gently into avocado hole with one egg yolk.
Keep on spooning into the hole with egg white until full. Repeat process with leftover avocado, egg white and egg yolk. Use pepper, sea salt, parsley, and chives to season each filled avocado.
In the preheated oven, gently position baking dish and bake for 15 minutes, until eggs are cooked. Sprinkle over avocado with bacon.

ALMOND & FRESH BERRY

Serv.: 4 | **Prep.:** 5m | **Cook:** 5m

Ingredients:
- ✓ 2 cups mixed fresh berries
- ✓ 1 teaspoon water (optional)
- ✓ 1/2 cup coconut milk
- ✓ 1 tablespoon ground cinnamon
- ✓ 1/2 cup almond meal

Directions: In a saucepan over medium heat, put berries. Cook, with cover about 5 minutes until berries soften and start to break apart. Put in a teaspoon of water if berries look dry when cooking. Take off from heat.
In a bowl, mix cinnamon and coconut milk.
Add berries to a bowl; pour coconut milk mixture on top of berries and scatter almond meal over.

PALEO BLUEBERRY CAST IRON PANCAKE

Serv.: 4 | **Prep.:** 10m | **Cook:** 23m

Ingredients:
- ✓ 3 tablespoons unsalted butter
- ✓ 8 eggs, room temperature
- ✓ 1 cup unsweetened vanilla-flavored almond milk
- ✓ 1/2 cup tapioca flour
- ✓ 2 tablespoons coconut flour
- ✓ 1 teaspoon lemon juice
- ✓ 1 teaspoon lemon zest
- ✓ 1/2 teaspoon sea salt
- ✓ 1 cup blueberries
- ✓ 2 tablespoons maple syrup, or to taste

Directions: Set oven to 400°F (200°C) for preheating.
Put butter in a cast iron pan and melt completely inside the oven as it preheats for 5 minutes.
In a bowl, mix well the milk and eggs; mix the coconut flour, lemon zest, sea salt, tapioca flour, and the lemon juice in. Mix well then add by folding the blueberries.

Get a kitchen towel or pot holder, then remove the pan from the oven. Coat the pan with melted butter using a pastry brush before pouring in the batter.
Put in heated oven and bake for 18-20 minutes until the top turns golden brown and the middle of the pancake becomes firm. Slice and top it with maple syrup before serving.

PALEO CARAMEL SAUCE

Serv.: 8 | **Prep.:** 5m | **Cook:** 4m

Ingredients:
- ✓ 1/2 cup honey
- ✓ 3 tablespoons unsweetened coconut cream

Directions: Whisk coconut cream and honey on medium high heat in a saucepan; cook, constantly mixing, till mixture reaches rolling boil. Put timer on 4 minutes. Mix caramel, scraping sides down constantly. Bubbles will be high yet airy.
Take saucepan off heat after 4 minutes exactly. Cool caramel for 3 minutes. It will thicken while cooling.

PALEO CHOCOLATE PEPPERMINT MINI DONUTS

Serv.: 12 | **Prep.:** 25m | **Cook:** 9m

Ingredients:
- ✓ 3/4 cup cassava flour (such as Otto's)
- ✓ 3 tablespoons unsweetened cocoa powder
- ✓ 1 teaspoon baking powder
- ✓ 1/4 teaspoon salt
- ✓ 1/4 cup butter, softened
- ✓ 2 tablespoons coconut sugar
- ✓ 3/4 cup full-fat coconut milk
- ✓ 6 tablespoons pure maple syrup
- ✓ 1 egg
- ✓ 1/2 teaspoon vanilla extract
- ✓ 1/2 teaspoon peppermint extract, or to taste
Chocolate Glaze:
- ✓ 1/2 cup semisweet chocolate chips
- ✓ 1 teaspoon coconut oil
- ✓ 1/4 teaspoon peppermint extract

✓ 1 peppermint candy cane, finely crushed

Directions: In a bowl, combine salt, cassava flour, baking powder, and cocoa powder.

In a big bowl, beat coconut sugar and butter together until fluffy using an electric mixer. Mix in half teaspoon peppermint extract, coconut milk, vanilla extract, maple syrup, and egg until well blended. Combine the butter mixture and flour mixture until evenly combined.

Prepare donut maker following the manufacturer's directions. With a clean and corner-cut ziplock bag or pastry bag, form batter into donuts.

Following the manufacturer's directions, bake for 4 m. Cool donuts in a rack for 15 m.

In a double broiler, melt and stir quarter teaspoon peppermint extract, chocolate chips, and coconut oil together until smooth. Transfer glaze in a shallow bowl. Submerge donut tops in glaze then in crushed candy canes; place the donuts back in the rack. Repeat process with leftover donuts.

PALEO SLOW COOKER TERIYAKI CHICKEN

Serv.: 8| **Prep.:** 15m | **Cook:** 2h30m

Ingredients:
✓ 3 pounds skinless, boneless chicken thighs
✓ 1/4 cup coconut aminos (soy-free seasoning sauce)
✓ 1/4 cup dry sherry
✓ 1/4 cup water
✓ 1 tablespoon rice wine vinegar
✓ 1 tablespoon toasted sesame oil
✓ 1 tablespoon grated fresh ginger
✓ 2 cloves garlic, minced
✓ 6 cups shredded bok choy
✓ 2 tablespoons sesame seeds (optional)

Directions: Put chicken thighs in a four-quart slow cooker.

Combine dry sherry, coconut aminos, water, sesame oil, rice wine vinegar, garlic and ginger in a bowl. Pour over the thighs.

Cook thighs on High for 2 1/2-3 hours, until softened.

Put them on a serving platter. Save the cooking juice from the slow cooker. Cover the thighs with aluminum foil so they remain warm.

Mix bok choy into the juices. Cover and leave them for 5 minutes, until wilted. Place bok choy on the serving platter. Pour some of the cooking juice on top. Throw away any remaining cooking juice. Top with sesame seeds.

PALEO SPAGHETTI SQUASH PRIMAVERA

Serv.: 6| **Prep.:** 30m | **Cook:** 48m

Ingredients:
✓ 1 spaghetti squash
✓ 2 tablespoons olive oil
✓ 1 large zucchini, chopped
✓ 1 teaspoon sea salt
✓ 1/2 teaspoon freshly ground black pepper to taste
✓ 1 red bell pepper, sliced
✓ 1 yellow onion, sliced
✓ 2 cloves garlic, chopped
✓ 2 cups trimmed fresh green beans
✓ 1 (14 ounce) can diced tomatoes
✓ 2 teaspoons Italian seasoning, or more to taste

Directions: Preheat an oven to 190°C/375°F. Poke 10 holes in spaghetti squash; put in baking pan.

In preheated oven, bake for 25 minutes till spaghetti squash is partially cooked and soft. Take out of oven; cool till easy to handle. Lower oven temperature to 175°C/350°F.

Halve spaghetti squash; seed. Use a fork to pull squash flesh from peel.

In braising pan, heat oil on medium high heat. Add pepper, salt and zucchini; mix and cook for 3-5 minutes till soft. Add garlic, onion and bell pepper; mix and cook for 3 minutes till flavors merge. Mix green beans in; cook for 2 minutes till bright green. Mix Italian seasoning and diced tomatoes into pan; simmer for 5 minutes till tomatoes are warm. Add spaghetti squash in; toss till combined. Use aluminum foil to cover.

In preheated oven, bake for 10 minutes tills spaghetti squash is tender.

PAN SEARED SCALLOPS

Serv.: 4| **Prep.:** 30m | **Cook:** 15m

Ingredients:
- ✓ 1/3 cup extra virgin olive oil
- ✓ 1 (2 ounce) can anchovy fillets, minced
- ✓ 1 pound large sea scallops
- ✓ 1 large red bell pepper, coarsely chopped
- ✓ 1 large orange bell pepper, coarsely chopped
- ✓ 1 red onion, coarsely chopped
- ✓ 2 cloves garlic, thinly sliced
- ✓ 1 teaspoon minced lime zest
- ✓ 1 1/2 teaspoons minced lemon zest
- ✓ 1 pinch kosher salt and pepper to taste
- ✓ 8 sprigs fresh parsley, for garnish

Directions: In a large skillet, bring minced anchovies and olive oil to medium-high heat, then stir while the oil is heating until no anchovies' lumps remain. When anchovies are sizzling, put in sea scallops, and cook for 2 minutes without disturbing the scallops.
In the meantime, combine lemon zest, lime zest, garlic, red onion, orange bell pepper and red bell pepper in a bowl; add pepper and salt to season. Scatter pepper mixture over scallops and keep cooking for another 2 minutes until scallops are browned. Flip scallops over, whisk pepper mixture, and keep cooking for 4-5 minutes more until scallops are browned on the opposite side. Decorate with parsley sprigs before serving.

SAUCE FOR ITALIAN PASTA

Serv.: 12| **Prep.:** 20m | **Cook:** 2h5m

Ingredients:
- ✓ 2 teaspoons olive oil, or as needed
- ✓ 1 sweet onion, diced
- ✓ 6 cloves garlic, minced
- ✓ 6 (28 ounce) cans Italian-style peeled tomatoes (such as Cento® San Marzano)
- ✓ 2 tablespoons chopped fresh oregano
- ✓ 1 tablespoon salt, or to taste
- ✓ 1 tablespoon ground black pepper, or to taste
- ✓ 10 leaves fresh basil

Directions: In a big pot, pour just enough olive oil to coat the bottom then put over medium heat. Cook and mix the sweet onion in the pot for 1 to 2 minutes until it releases some moisture. Mix garlic with the onion then cook for a minute more. Immediately take the pot away from the heat.
In a big food mill, use medium holes to process the tomatoes and grind directly into the pot. Over medium-low heat, let the tomato mixture come to a light simmer; season it using pepper, salt and oregano. Let it simmer, stirring regularly, for an hour.
Mix basil leaves into the sauce. Allow it to simmer, stirring regularly again, for another hour.

PAPRIKA CHICKEN

Serv.: 6| **Prep.:** 10m | **Cook:** 40m

Ingredients:
- ✓ 6 skinless, boneless chicken breasts
- ✓ Ground black pepper to taste
- ✓ 1 pinch garlic powder
- ✓ 1 teaspoon poultry seasoning
- ✓ 2 teaspoons paprika

Directions: Preheat an oven to 190°C/375°F; grease the 9x13-in. baking dish lightly.
Arrange the chicken breasts into the baking dish, side by side. Sprinkle on the paprika, poultry seasoning, garlic powder and ground black pepper to season the chicken breasts. In preheated oven, bake the breasts till juices are clear and the meat is not pink on the inside, about 40-50 minutes. Check frequently; if chicken begins to stick to dish, add a little water.

PARCHMENT BAKED SALMON

Serv.: 2| **Prep.:** 15m | **Cook:** 25m

Ingredients:
- ✓ 1 (8 ounce) salmon fillet
- ✓ Salt and ground black pepper to taste
- ✓ 1/4 cup chopped basil leaves

- ✓ Olive oil cooking spray
- ✓ 1 lemon, thinly sliced

Directions: Put the rack in the lowest position in the oven and preheat to 400°F (200°C).

In the middle of a large piece of parchment paper, arrange salmon fillet with skin side down; use black pepper and salt to season. Use a sharp knife to make 2 3-inch slits on the fish body. Use chopped basil leaves to stuff into the slits. Use cooking spray to coat the fillet and top with lemon slices.

Take the edges of the parchment paper and fold over the fish a couple of times to secure into an airtight packet. Put it onto the baking sheet.

Put the fish on the bottom rack and bake for 25 minutes until the meat turns opaque and pink with lightly darker pink color in the interior and salmon can be easily flaked. Insert an instant-read meat thermometer into the thickest part of the fillet. Take out when it reaches 145°F (65°C). Open the parchment paper and discard lemon slices before serving.

PASTA SAUCE WITH ITALIAN SAUSAGE

Serv.: 6 | **Prep.:** 30m | **Cook:** 1h

Ingredients:
- ✓ 1 pound Italian sausage links
- ✓ 1/2 pound lean ground beef
- ✓ 1 tablespoon olive oil
- ✓ 1 onion, chopped
- ✓ 1 clove garlic, chopped
- ✓ 1 (16 ounce) can canned tomatoes
- ✓ 1 (15 ounce) can canned tomato sauce
- ✓ 1 teaspoon salt
- ✓ 1/4 teaspoon ground black pepper
- ✓ 1 teaspoon dried basil
- ✓ 1 teaspoon dried oregano
- ✓ 1 bay leaf

Directions: Remove casings from sausage links; cut into 1/2 in. slices. Place a large skillet on medium heat, brown sausages for around 10 minutes; remove; set aside.

Place a large skillet on medium heat, heat onion, garlic, olive oil and ground beef till meat is nicely browned; strain.

Add in tomato sauce and tomatoes; combine in cooked sausage, bay leaf, oregano, basil, ground black pepper and salt. Simmer without a cover while stirring from time to time for 1 hour.

Allow a large pot of slightly salted water to boil. Include in pasta; cook till al dente, or for 8-10 minutes; strain.

Combine cooked sauce with hot pasta; discard bay leaf from the sauce before serving.

PEACH AND BERRY SALAD

Serv.: 4 | **Prep.:** 15m | **Cook:** 5m

Ingredients:
- ✓ 3 fresh peaches
- ✓ 2 1/2 pints blackberries
- ✓ 1 pint strawberries, hulled and sliced
- ✓ 1/4 cup honey
- ✓ 1/2 teaspoon ground cardamom

Directions: Boil water in a medium pot. Place in peaches and blanch for 30 seconds. Drain and move to a medium bowl. Add cold water to cover and allow to cool. Drain and peel the peaches then slice.

Combine cardamom, honey, strawberries, blackberries and peaches in a medium bowl. Toss together and store in the fridge.

PEAR BRAISED PORK TENDERLOIN

Serv.: 4 | **Prep.:** 30m | **Cook:** 45m

Ingredients:
- ✓ 1 ripe pear, cored and coarsely chopped
- ✓ 1 clove garlic, pressed
- ✓ 3/4 cup extra-virgin olive oil
- ✓ 1/2 cup dry white wine
- ✓ 1/2 teaspoon minced rosemary
- ✓ 1 (1 1/2 pound) pork tenderloin, cut in half
- ✓ 1 teaspoon sea salt
- ✓ 1 teaspoon ground mixed peppercorns
- ✓ 5 pearl onions, peeled and chopped

Directions: Preheat an oven to 190 °C or 375 °F. Crush together rosemary, white wine, olive oil, garlic and soft pear. Add pepper and salt into pork to taste, and put into a glass 10x10-inch baking dish. Top pork with pear mixture and scatter chopped onion over. Put aluminum foil on baking dish to cover.

In the prepped oven, bake for approximately 45 minutes, till inner heat of pork attains 63 °C or 145 °F once taken using meat thermometer.

PEPPERONI MEATZA

Serv.: 6 | **Prep.:** 30m | **Cook:** 15m

Ingredients:
- ✓ 1 tablespoon salt
- ✓ 1 teaspoon caraway seeds (optional)
- ✓ 1 teaspoon dried oregano
- ✓ 1 teaspoon garlic salt
- ✓ 1 teaspoon ground black pepper
- ✓ 1 teaspoon red pepper flakes, or to taste (optional)
- ✓ 2 pounds extra lean ground beef
- ✓ 2 eggs
- ✓ 1/2 cup grated Parmesan cheese
- ✓ 1 (12 ounce) package shredded mozzarella cheese
- ✓ 1 cup tomato sauce
- ✓ 1 (3.5 ounce) package sliced pepperoni, or to taste

Directions: Start preheating the oven at 450°F (230°C).

Combine crushed red pepper flakes, ground black pepper, garlic salt, oregano, caraway seeds, and salt in a small bowl.

In a mixing bowl, mix eggs and ground beef until well incorporated. Add seasoning mixture and Parmesan cheese to beef; blend. In a 12x17-inch pan, press the ground beef mixture and spread out evenly.

Bake in the prepared oven for about 10 minutes until meat is not pink anymore. Drain the grease. Place the oven rack about 6 inches from the heat source and start to heat the oven's broiler.

Scatter 1/3 of the mozzarella cheese over the baked meat, followed by tomato sauce in a level layer. Scatter again 1/3 of the mozzarella cheese over the sauce and place slices of pepperoni on top. Sprinkle pizza with the leftover mozzarella cheese.

Broil for 3 to 5 minutes until cheese melts, bubbles, and turns to lightly brown.

PERFECT RIB ROAST

Serv.: 6 | **Prep.:** 30m | **Cook:** 1h45m

Ingredients:
- ✓ 1 1/2 teaspoons lemon-pepper seasoning
- ✓ 1 1/2 teaspoons paprika
- ✓ 3/4 teaspoon garlic salt
- ✓ 1/2 teaspoon dried rosemary, crushed
- ✓ 1/2 teaspoon cayenne pepper
- ✓ 1 (4 pound) boneless beef rib roast

Directions: Set an oven at 175°C (350°F) to preheat.

Mix cayenne pepper, rosemary, garlic salt, paprika, and lemon-pepper seasoning in a small dish. Rub all over the whole roast.

Arrange the roast on a roasting rack with the fat side up inside a shallow roasting pan.

In the preheated oven, bake for 1 hour and 40 minutes, or until the roast reaches at least 63°C (145°F) for medium-rare, or your desired degree of doneness. Medium is ideal: 70°C (160°F). Before carving into thin slices, allow the roast to rest for 10-15 minutes.

CONCLUSION

Thank you again for reading "Paleo Diet for Family"!

I hope you enjoyed reading my book.

Now all you have to do is try making the recipes you like best. You can try to create them as they are listed or make a few small variations in quantities or ingredients.

You will then have the opportunity to experiment with so many recipes for the whole family!

Our health depends on the quality of our food and the PALEO DIET will help you regain energy and health!

I suggest always consulting a nutritionist to figure out which diet is best for you.

Good luck!

Tess Connors

CPSIA information can be obtained
at www.ICGtesting.com
Printed in the USA
BVHW011353210621
610125BV00009B/2547